THE DARK ART OF LIFE MASTERY

THE DARK ART OF
LIFE MASTERY

YOUR LIFE, YOUR WAY, RIGHT HERE, RIGHT NOW

HUSSEIN HALLAK

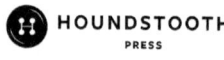
HOUNDSTOOTH
PRESS

COPYRIGHT © 2025 HUSSEIN HALLAK
All rights reserved.

THE DARK ART OF LIFE MASTERY
Your Life, Your Way, Right Here, Right Now

FIRST EDITION

ISBN   978-1-5445-4587-5   *Hardcover*
           978-1-5445-4586-8   *Paperback*
           978-1-5445-4588-2   *Ebook*

This work is licensed under the Creative Commons Attribution-ShareAlike 4.0 International License. To view a copy of this license, visit http://creativecommons.org/licenses/by-sa/4.0/ or send a letter to Creative Commons, PO Box 1866, Mountain View, CA 94042, USA.

You are free to:

Share—copy and redistribute the material in any medium or format.

Adapt—remix, transform, and build upon the material for any purpose, even commercially.

The licensor cannot revoke these freedoms as long as you follow the license terms.

Under the following terms:

Attribution—You must give appropriate credit, provide a link to the license, and indicate if changes were made. You may do so in any reasonable manner, but not in any way that suggests the licensor endorses you or your use.

ShareAlike—If you remix, transform, or build upon the material, you must distribute your contributions under the same license as the original.

No additional restrictions—You may not apply legal terms or technological measures that legally restrict others from doing anything the license permits.

Notices:

You do not have to comply with the license for elements of the material in the public domain or where your use is permitted by an applicable exception or limitation.

No warranties are given. The license may not give you all of the permissions necessary for your intended use. For example, other rights such as publicity, privacy, or moral rights may limit how you use the material.

CONTENTS

REWIND	9
(UNTITLED)	15
TIME IS THE KEY	21
THEN YOU DIE	27
LET GO	31
CAPTAIN ON DECK	37
MASTER	41
AT THE HELM	45
TAKE IT IN	51
HOLD ON	55
YOU	59
SPLIT SECOND	63
SCANNING	67
MIND THE GAP	71
SNAP OUT OF IT	75
MIND YOUR THOUGHTS	81
RIGHT HERE. RIGHT NOW.	87
GO BIG	93

TEMPORARY JOYS	99
GO HOME	103
THERE'S TIME	107
SOMEDAY	113
THE ONE THING	119
A FUTURE	125
COMPASS	129
NORTH	135
MINDSET	141
SLOW IT DOWN	147
ONLY HUMAN	153
THE FALL	157
SURRENDER	163
RECOVER	167
FLOW	171
STEP INTO IT	175
80/20	179
RECHARGE AT 80	185
SAY NO	193
NO IS A YES	199
TEST	205
CURB YOUR ENTHUSIASM	209
START WITH 20	213
JAM ON IT	219
UNSTOPPABLE	225
FASTER. EASIER. BETTER.	229
WHAT IS ENOUGH?	233
CHOICE	239
THIS BOOK IS IMPOSSIBLE	245
ABOUT THE AUTHOR	251

REWIND

PUT ON YOUR MASTERY SUNGLASSES

—JOEL MARK HARRIS

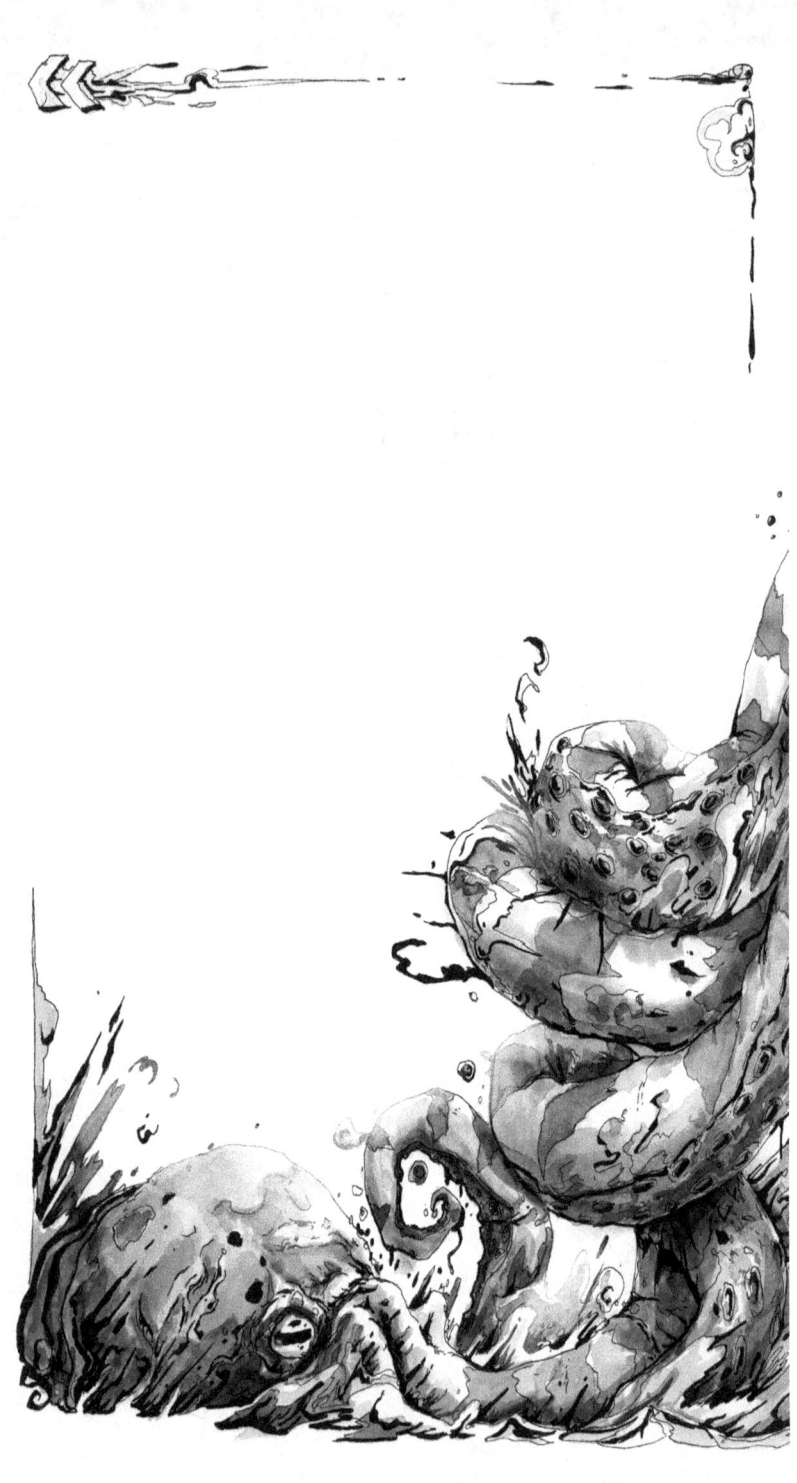

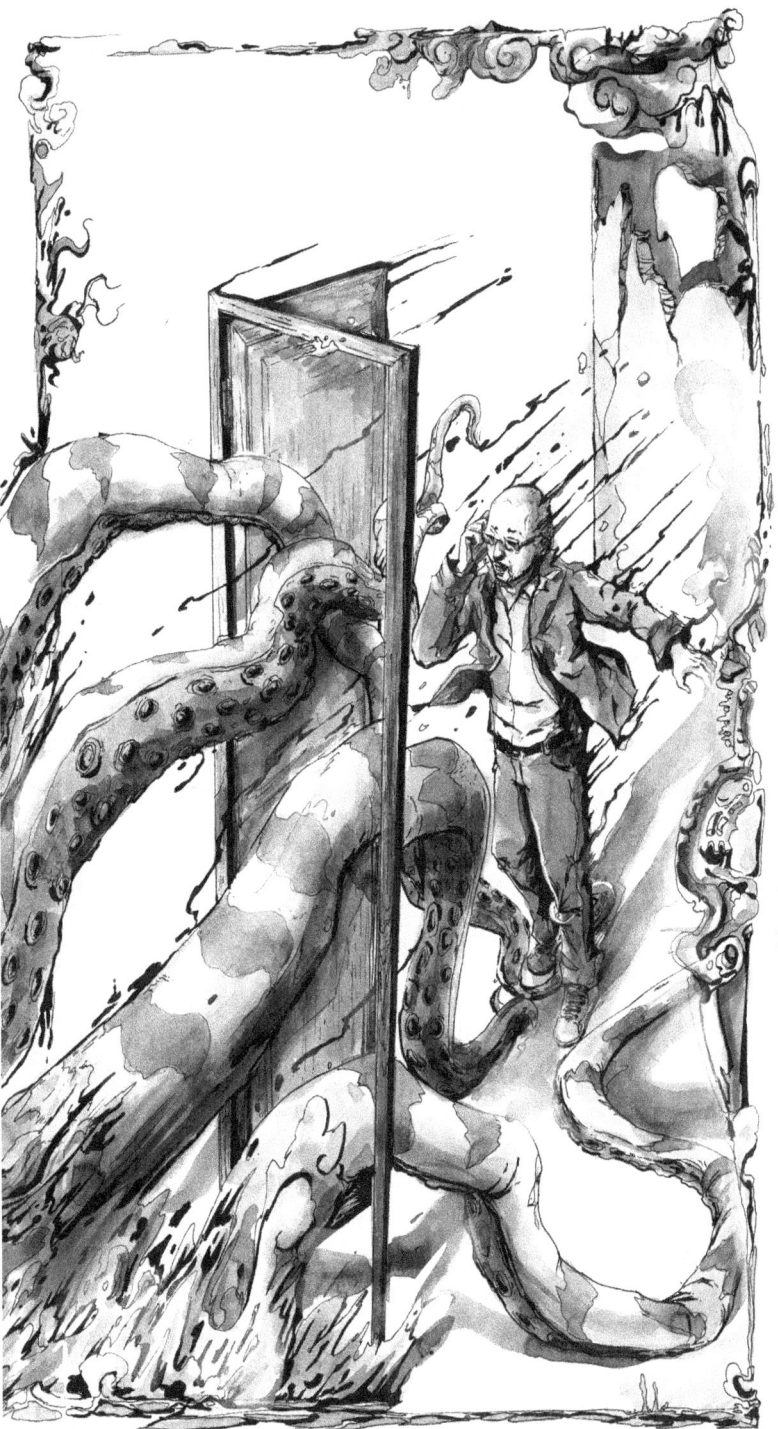

There isn't anything here you don't already know or couldn't discover for yourself.

Hussein's writing is as easy as putting on a pair of sunglasses.

Sunglasses aren't right or wrong; they just allow you to see things differently based upon the environment surrounding you.

YOU'LL FIND THIS BOOK PACKS A PUNCH WITH EVERY WORD, EVERY SENTENCE, AND EVERY PARAGRAPH.

Nothing is wasted.

As a result, this book won't take you long to consume; however, it will take a lifetime to master.

And that is how it should be.

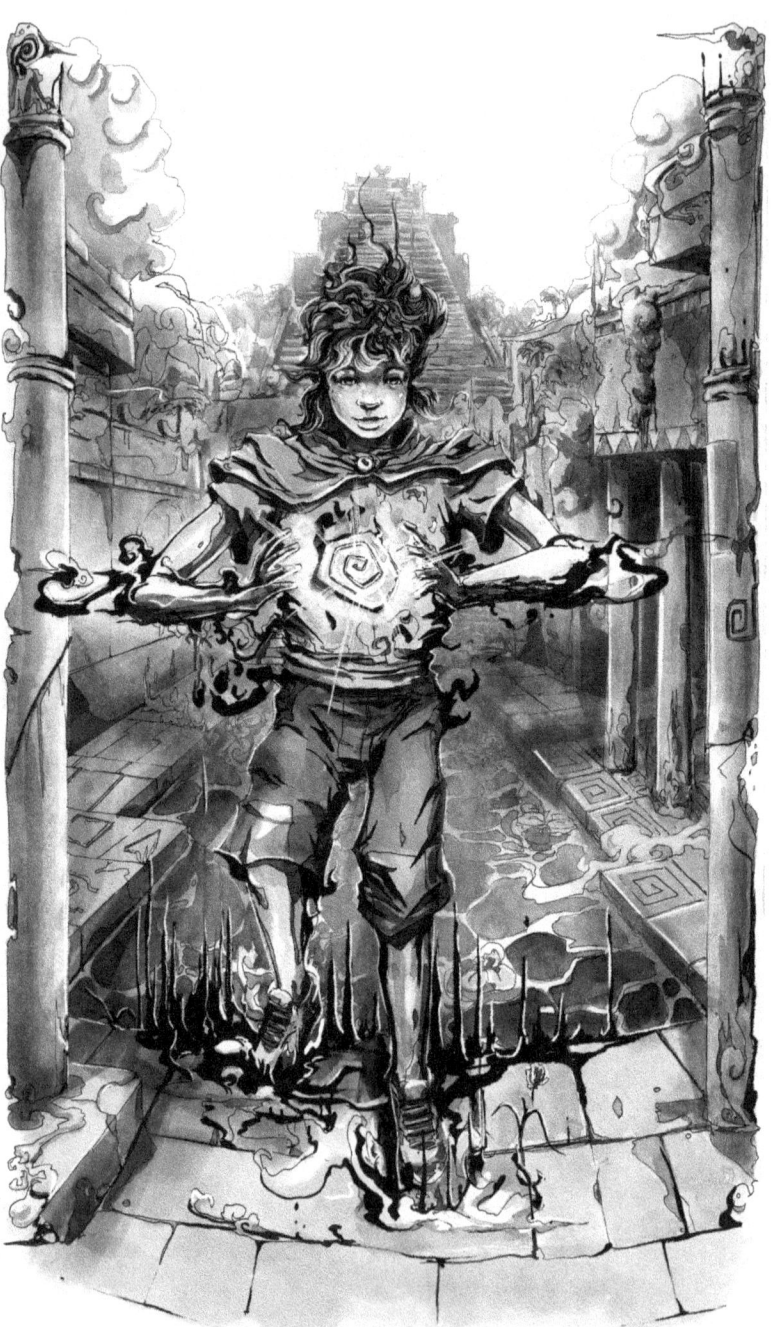

GROWING UP IN SYRIA IN THE 1980S, MY DAY IS A BLUR—FINDING ANYTHING TO KEEP BUSY TILL THE MOST IMPORTANT HOUR OF THE DAY COMES.

It's almost 4:00 p.m. My mom is trying hard to get us unstuck from the TV, but the moment she goes to the kitchen, we're glued back to the screen, close enough to see the three colored pixels.

It's the latest episode of *The Adventures of Pepero*. We sing along with the theme song. We can't wait to find out what's going to happen next.

We've been following Pepero for months now. A young boy living in the Andes, Pepero sets off on a journey to find his father, who's gone missing while on a quest to find Eldorado, a secret city made entirely out of gold where no one ever goes hungry.

On his remarkable journey into the unknown, danger is at every turn. We are right there with Pepero, cheering him on, and shouting down his powerful enemies who will stop at nothing to get to Eldorado first.

This ten-year-old kid is all of us. Even when challenged beyond what anyone can withstand, his love for his father keeps him going. His journey continues with the help of a golden eagle, a majestic white horse, and loyal friends he makes along the way.

After many adventures, the final episode is here. We are jumping up and down as we sing the theme song one last time.

Yes! Pepero finds his father and the lost city of Eldorado.

We are on the couches cheering like crazy.

The legends are true. Eldorado is beyond what anyone could imagine. Everything is made of gold, everyone is well dressed and happy, kids are playing, and feasts are everywhere.

Mom comes screaming to get us off the furniture before we break something.

Wait! What?! It's not over yet!

Pepero discovers his journey has just begun, and the search for Eldorado doesn't end with finding the city.

Along with his friends, they uncover a plot to take over Eldorado. They manage to stop their enemies, and save the king's life and the lives of his son and daughter.

The king holds a ceremony that brings all of Eldorado together to honor Pepero and his friends. He offers Pepero all the gold and precious stones he can carry back to his village.

Pepero remembers the wise words of his dying grandfather: "I believe in you, my son. You will reach Eldorado. But, careful not to let the gold blind you. Pepero, you must bring back the treasure of the forefathers to save our people."

Pepero declines the king's offer and asks for the treasure of the forefathers.

The king smiles and invites Pepero to a massive, heavily guarded doorway. They walk through and stand at the edge of never-ending fields of golden corn. Pepero gasps.

The king whispers, "This is the true treasure our forefathers left us. The gold is just a facade to trick thieves and stop them from finding our true source of wealth."

The king signals his guards to bring bags of corn seeds for Pepero and his friends.

The king hands the corn to Pepero and says, "Take these seeds to help your people, but remember these seeds will not grow on their own. What will really help your people is the courage, hard work, compassion, and wisdom which got you and your friends to Eldorado."

Pepero heads back to his village with the seeds, fulfilling his destiny as the hero and savior of his people. And his search for Eldorado finally ends with finding it within himself.

Your journey to success and mastery of anything in life is much like Pepero's search for Eldorado, an outer world journey to find your inner world treasure.

YOUR ELDORADO IS WAITING.

TIME IS THE KEY

THE STUFF YOUR LIFE IS MADE OF

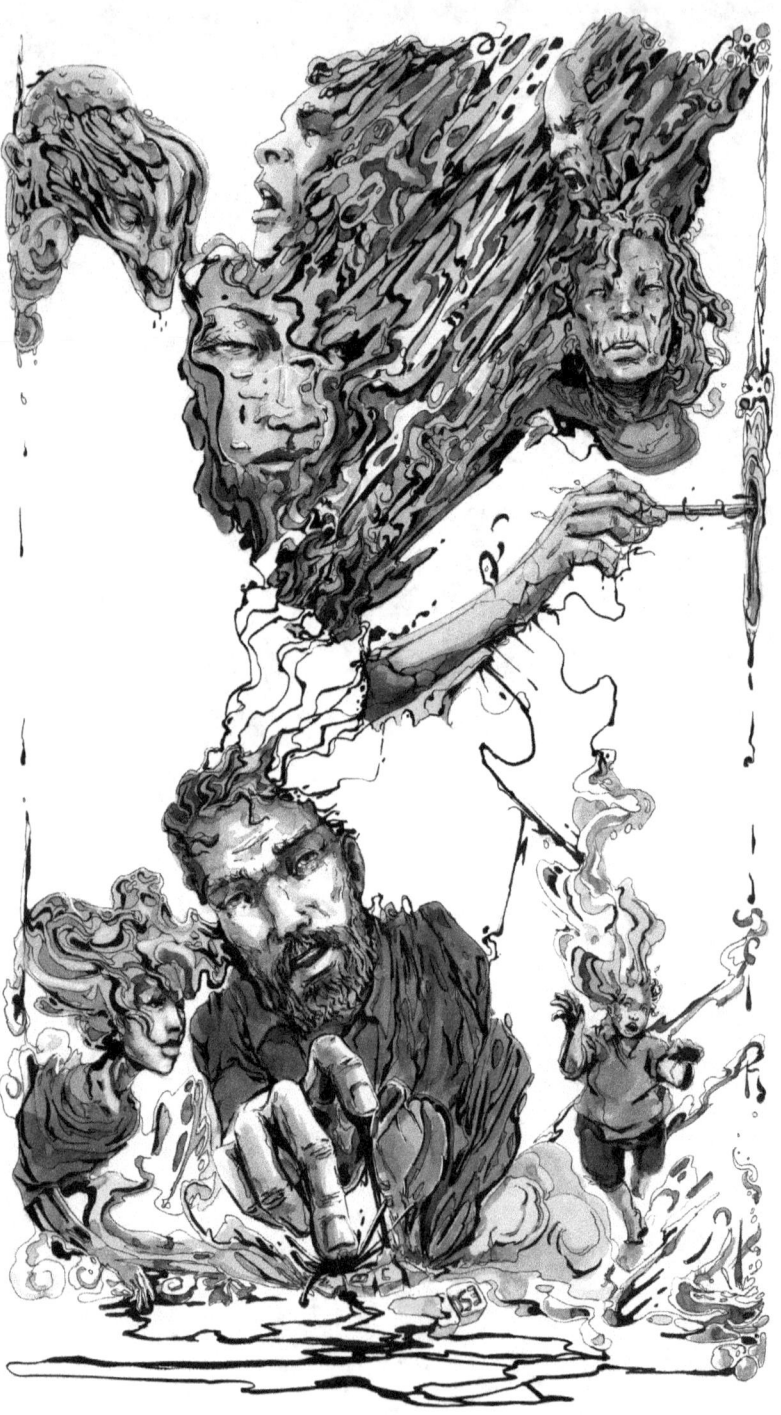

It's midweek, on a Wednesday afternoon.

A GLORIOUS DAY AT THE START OF THE MONTH. YOU'RE FEELING PRETTY GOOD ABOUT YOURSELF AND YOU'VE GOT EVERYTHING UNDER CONTROL.

You receive an email from *your old boss*, inviting you to work on a promising project that you started together a while back.

One of *your tweets* is trending! You're getting dozens of notifications, and you feel the need to jump into the conversation.

Your significant other suggests spending a few hours on the beach. You've been spending way too much time at the office, and he misses you.

The long-awaited sequel to *your favorite movie* of all time just dropped, and you just have to get the premiere tickets before they run out.

Your daughter bursts into your home office and won't leave until you pet her cat and play UNO with her!

It's tax season, and you must get *your financials* in order. Something you've been avoiding and postponing all year!

Some new deals came through. You're excited as you've been working on them for what seems to be forever. Now, along with *your team*, you have some new deadlines to fulfill.

The phone rings. You get the devastating news of a distant family member passing away, and *your mom* says you need to be at the funeral next week.

You check *your email* and find a request for an interview from the number one podcast in your industry. They need your confirmation within the hour.

It's Thursday evening two weeks later. The more you do, the more *your to-do list* expands and grows. You feel drained and in need of some time off to recover and recharge.

If you really break it down, life is a collection of demands on your time.

THEN YOU DIE

YOU HAVE NO IDEA WHEN

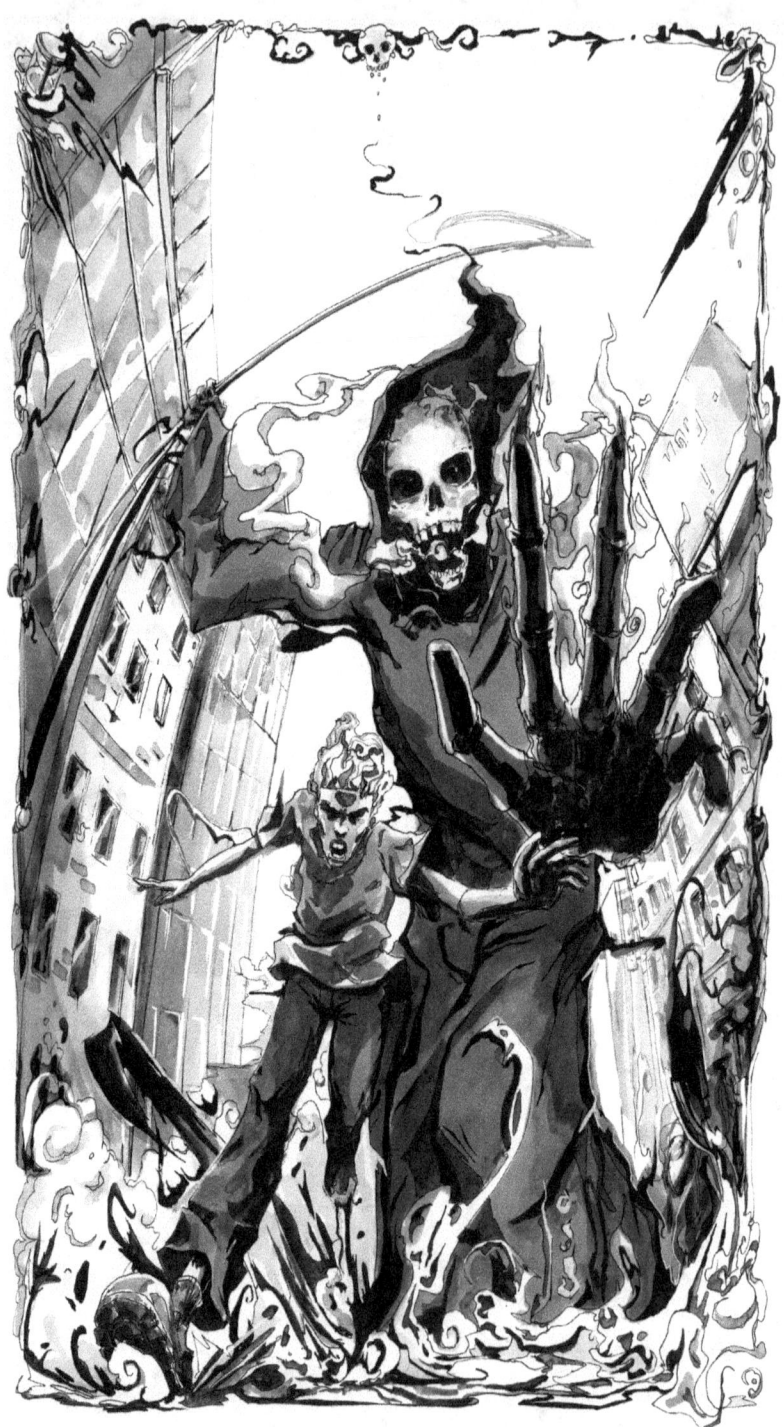

Worldwide, the average life expectancy at birth is 69 years.

That's 828 months, 3,598 weeks, 25,185 days, 6,044,240 hours, or 36,266,396 minutes, forever passing no matter who you are or what you plan to do with your life.

YOU CAN'T STOP LIFE, CAN'T SLOW IT DOWN, AND YOU CAN'T HOLD ON TO IT. BUT YOU CAN MASTER IT.

LET GO

LIFE DOESN'T ASK FOR PERMISSION

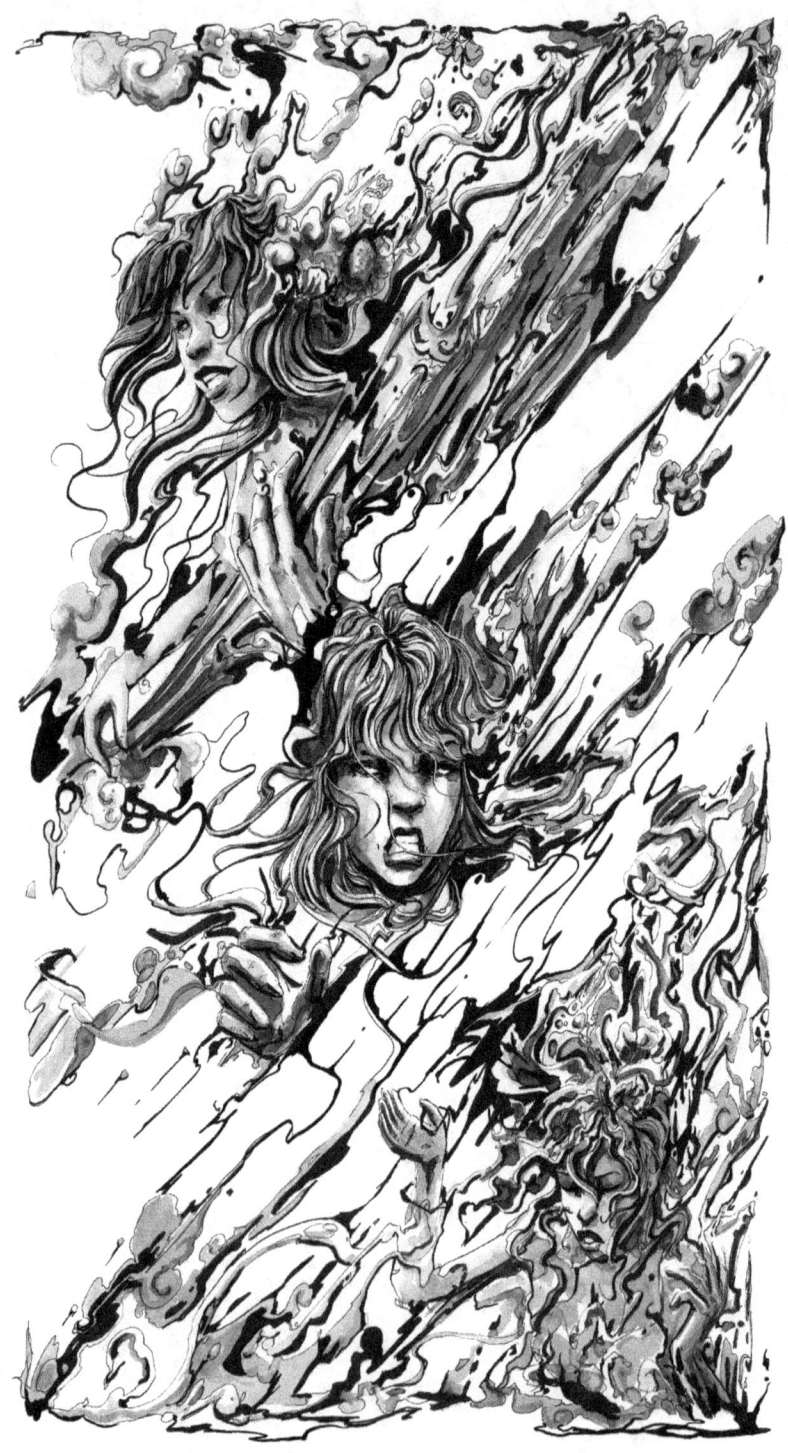

Life just happens. Things take place mostly with complete disregard to your well-thought-out plans and your New Year resolution to "once and for all, take charge of your life and become the master of your destiny."

However, life is made up of things you love, things you hate, and things you just have to deal with regardless of how you feel.

Let's say you:

- love playing the guitar, working on a passion project, or spending time with friends traveling the world
- hate going to the dentist for a regular checkup and avoid long and meaningless meetings like they are the plague
- can't be bothered to renew your car insurance or wait for the plumber to come and fix a leaking pipe

Surely as someone who's fully in control of your life, you will choose to do things you love like playing the guitar and traveling with friends, postponing your visit to the dentist and ignoring renewing your car insurance, right?!

However, life doesn't care.

The next time your tooth aches while practicing your favorite new tune, you'll quickly drop your guitar, call and beg the dentist for an early appointment, and then wait in pain for a friend to drive you because your car has no insurance.

So much for being in control!

Like the rest of us, you have the illusion of control that helps you go through life without freaking out.

IN REALITY, DEEP INSIDE, YOU KNOW YOU DON'T CONTROL SHIT.

Yes, you are holding that pot and pouring yourself a delicious, perfectly prepared cup of coffee on a morning that couldn't be more amazing.

You are on top of the world.

What you don't know is there's a call finding its way to you to knock you off of your imaginary throne of control and turn this day into one from hell.

The time has come to let the illusion go, renounce the throne, and seek your forefathers' treasure.

EMBRACE YOUR TRUE PURPOSE, CLAIM YOUR BIRTHRIGHT, AND TAKE YOUR PLACE AT THE HELM.

CAPTAIN ON DECK

SOMETIMES IN THE MIDDLE OF NOWHERE, YOU FIND YOURSELF

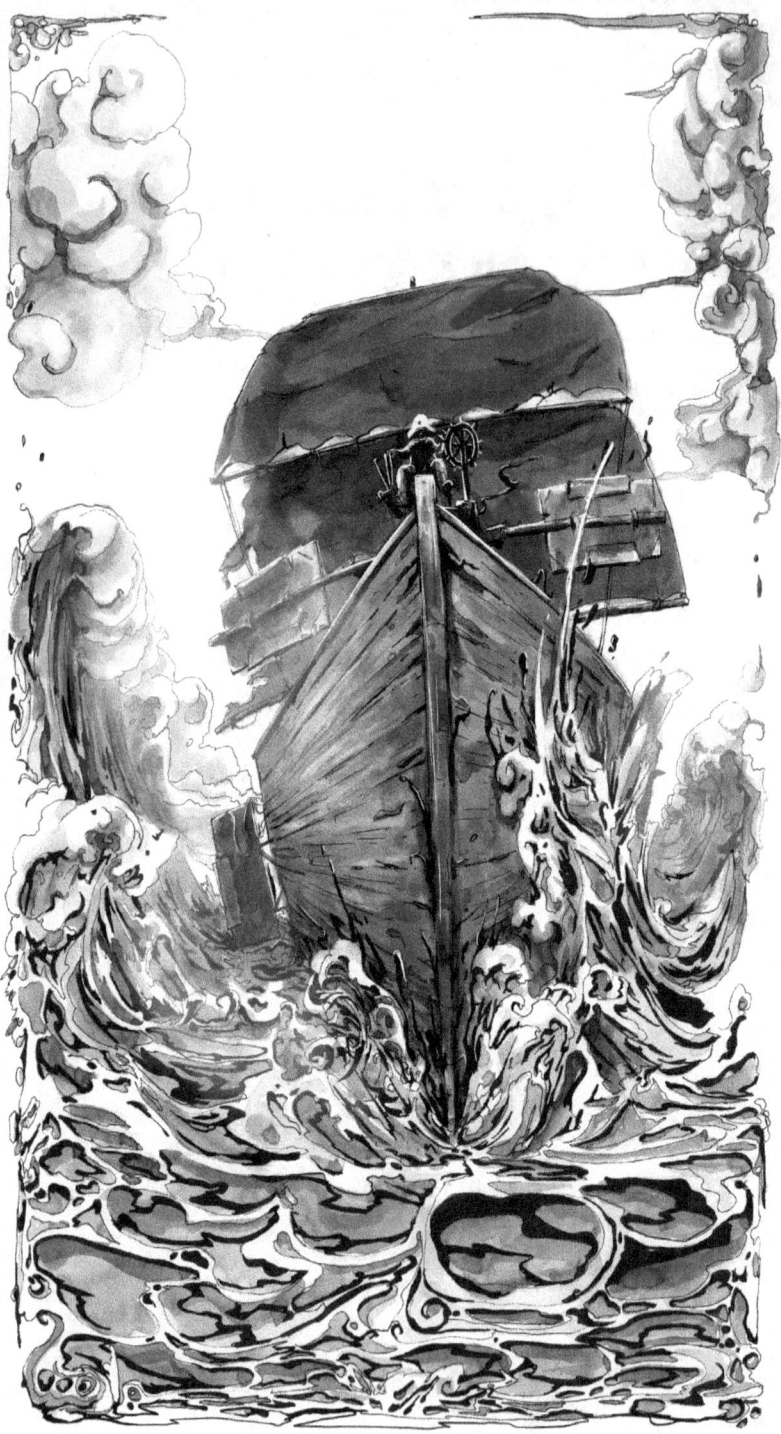

You're on a ship. Unrelenting wind and angry waves attack you from every direction.

No stars to guide you home. No safe harbor over the horizon. No clear destination.

YOU'RE LOST IN THE SEA OF LIFE—CALM AND SERENE ONE MOMENT, WILD AND UNFORGIVING THE NEXT.

As king, high up in your imaginary throne of control, you proclaim your dominion over the elements, give orders to move forward, command the sea to settle down, and ask the wind to take you to your destination.

BUT YOU'RE NOT KING. YOU'RE A CAPTAIN.

Step on deck and take the fucking wheel.

MASTER

**THE SEA OWES
YOU NOTHING**

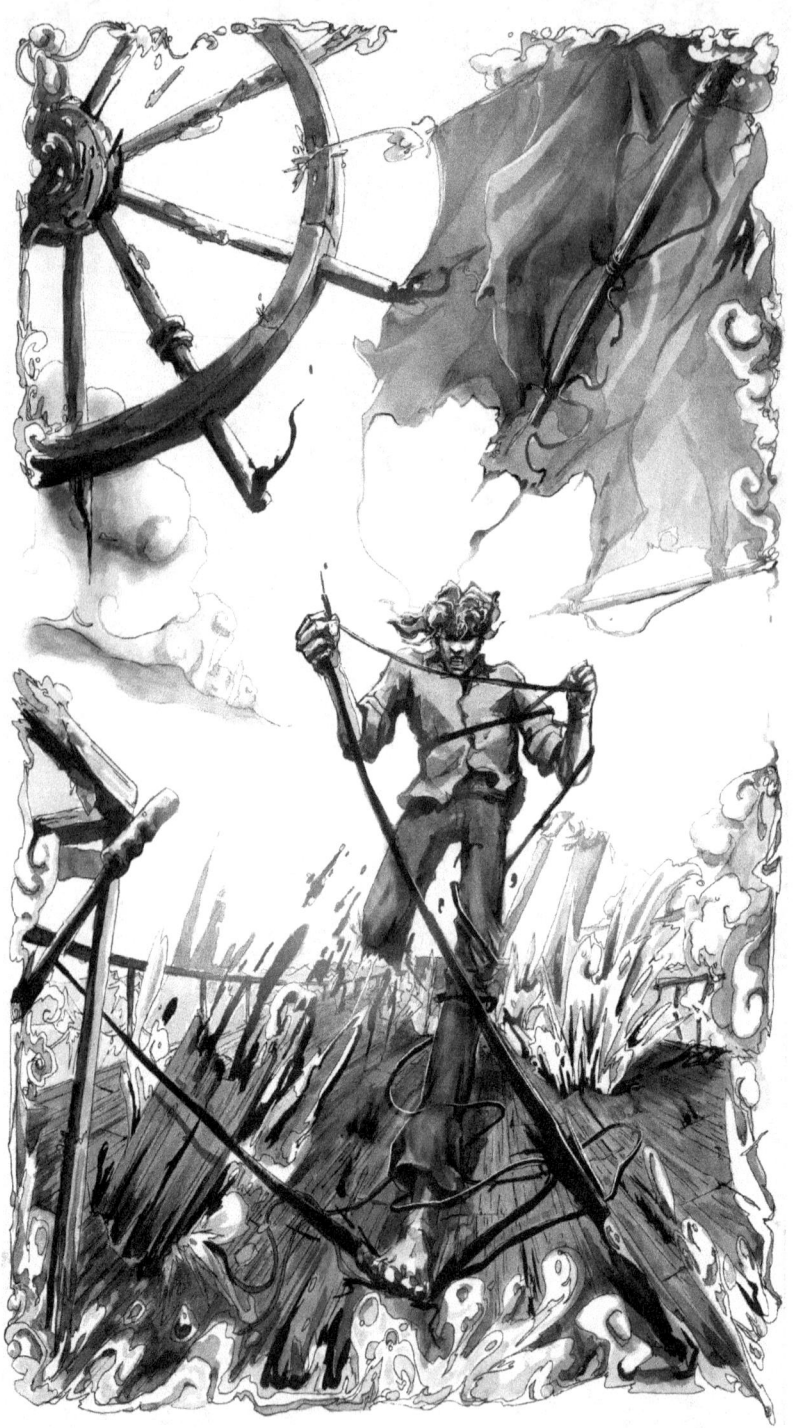

With your first step on the deck—even if you are the most capable captain to ever steer a ship—the sea of life doesn't give a shit. It owes you nothing.

It will keep on keeping on with complete disregard for you and your wishes, desires, or earned accolades from years of navigating its treacherous waters.

No guarantees, no assurances, and no promises.

YOUR FIRST LESSON IN MASTERY IS TO EXPECT NOTHING AND EXPECT EVERYTHING.

The sea of life might give you safe passage to your desired destination, and might just as well throw everything it has at you.

The sooner you put your hands on the wheel, start navigating the demands life places on you, and overcome the challenges it throws at you, the sooner you build the skills you need to navigate the demands it will place on you and overcome the challenges it will throw at you.

It's the very real, unrelenting, never-ending circle that's your life.

Then you die!

AT THE HELM

BECAUSE YOU MUST

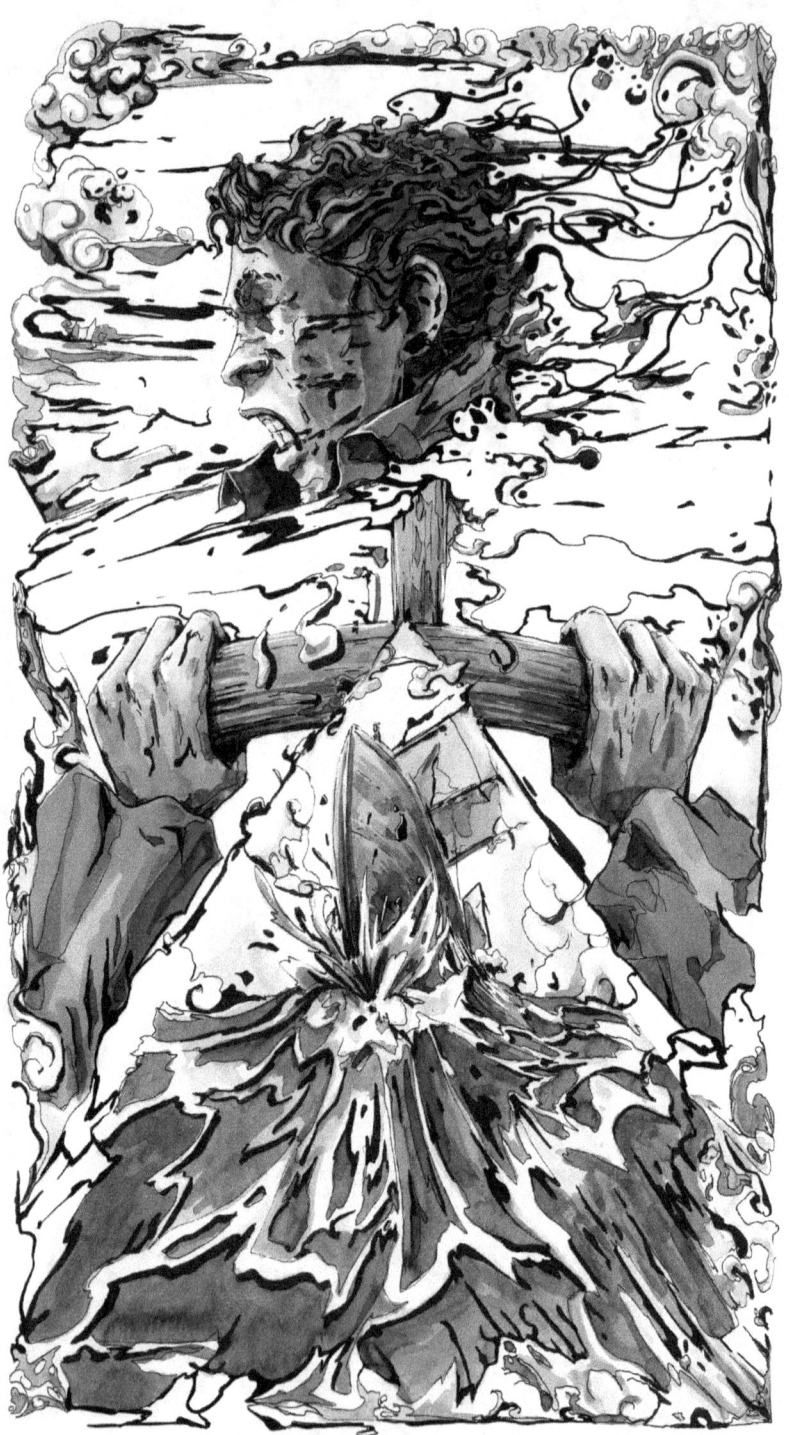

You stand.

Unless your ship breaks into little pieces, you stand.

Unless the current pulls you into the darkness of the unknown, you stand.

Hands tightly gripping the wheel, feet apart, eyes on the next destination, heart poised, lips slightly bent, as every cell celebrates the moment with every breath you take.

YOU STAND AT THE HELM. BECAUSE YOU CHOOSE TO.

You stand at the helm.

Because you can.

You stand at the helm.

Because you must.

You stand at the helm.

Because it's your birthright.

You stand at the helm.

Because you demand more.

YOU STAND AT THE HELM. BECAUSE IT'S WHO YOU ARE. YOU STAND AT THE HELM. UNSTOPPABLE.

TAKE IT IN

IT'S YOUR MOMENT

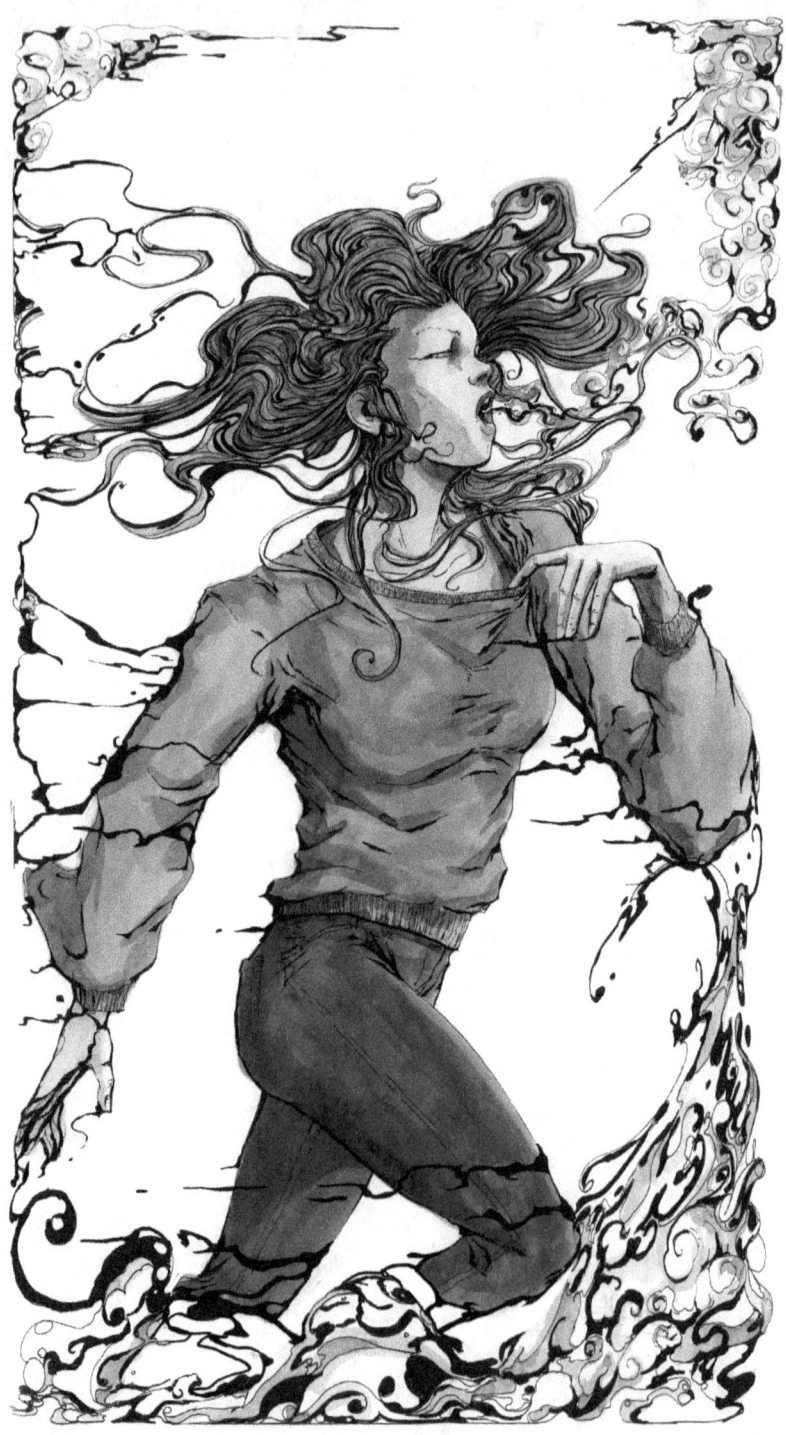

Take a breath.

Let it out.

Take another.

Let it out.

Feel it going in…and out of your body.

Anchor yourself in the moment.

Feel your body.

Feel every sensation as you breathe in…and out.

When ready, keep going.

HOLD ON

YOU CAN CLOSE YOUR EYES, BUT YOU CAN'T UNSEE

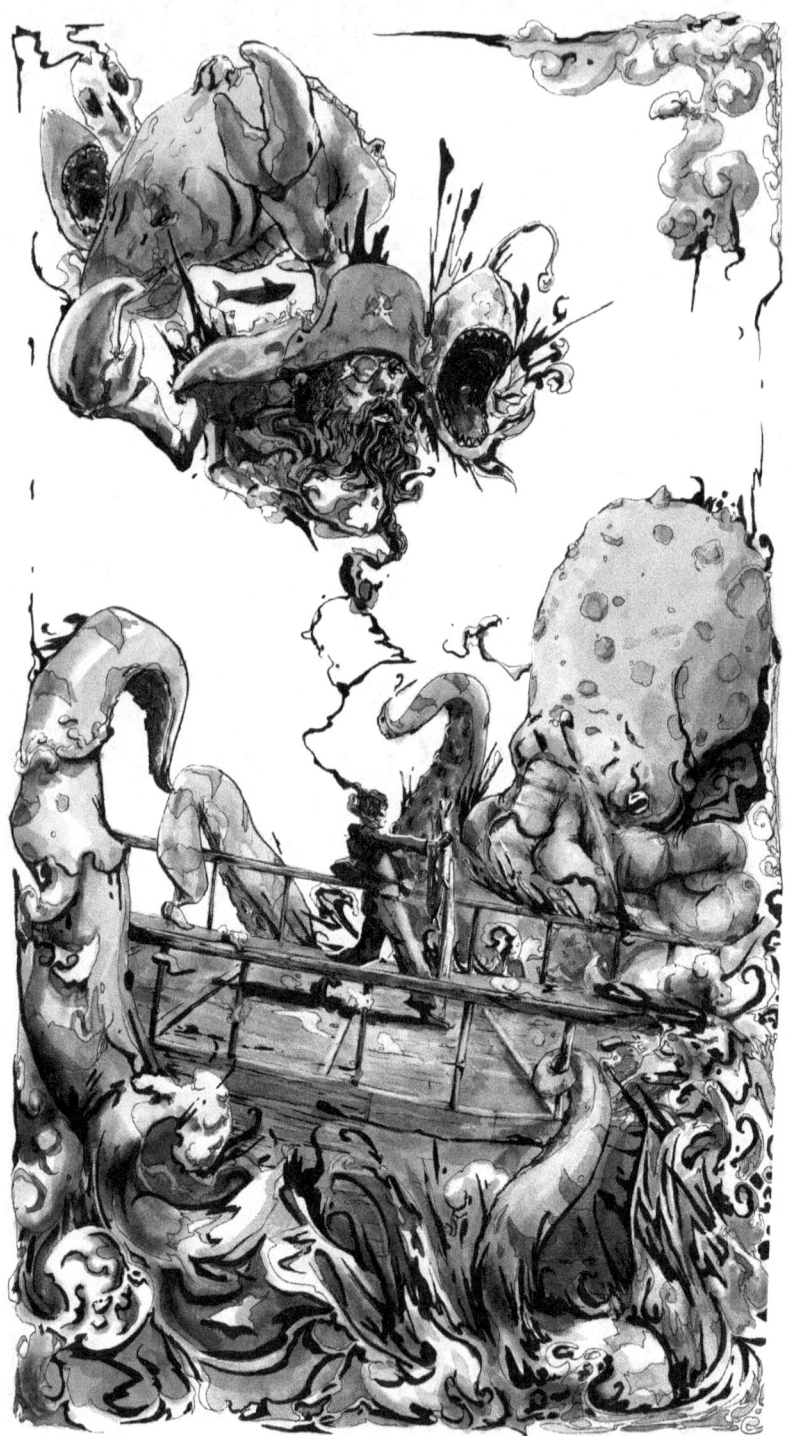

You stand at the helm.

Poised and determined as adventure awaits.

Unknowable.

Inevitable.

Burdened with stories of evil sea monsters, ruthless pirates, starvation, mutiny, and falling off the edge of the world.

You stand at the helm. You hold on tightly.

The promise of your destination and a remarkable life journey in front of you.

BEHIND YOU, MILLENNIA OF BELIEFS, HISTORY, AND LIFE EXPERIENCES SHAPE YOUR EVERY THOUGHT.

You can't unsee it.

You can't unthink it.

YOU

NEVER THE PASSIVE OBSERVER

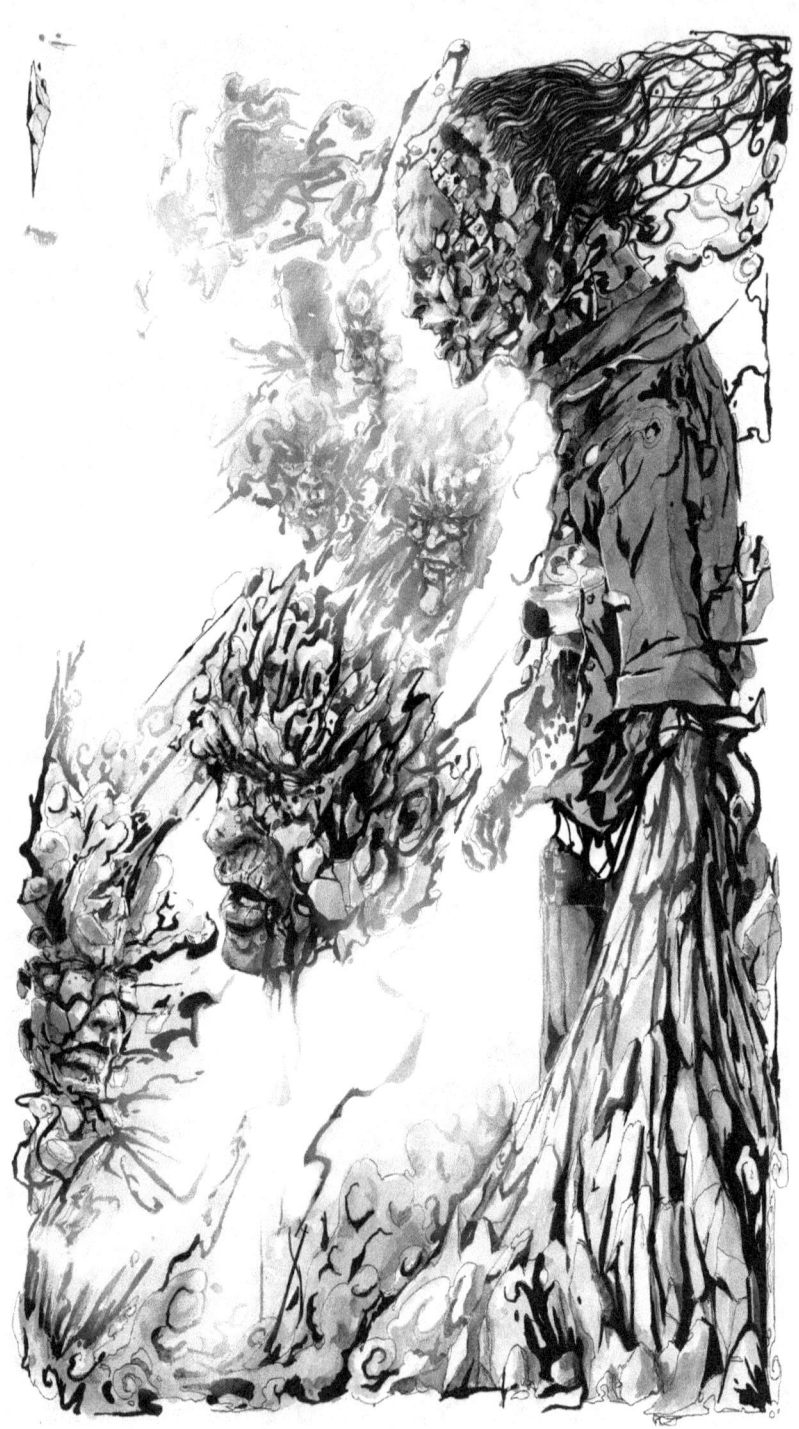

An amalgamation of your past, future, and present, you don't see things for what they really are.

You can't.

YOUR EXPERIENCE IS NOT A RESULT OF YOUR REALITY, BUT OF HOW YOU PERCEIVE THAT REALITY.

The sum of your thoughts, feelings, and actions.

Beliefs.

History.

Life.

Everything that makes you who you are shapes your reality and your perception of it.

BUILT TO FIND, CONSTRUCT, AND UTILIZE PATTERNS EVEN WHEN ALL YOU HAVE IS RANDOM, DISCONNECTED INFORMATION. YOU CONNECT THE DOTS, PIECE TOGETHER STORIES, AND SELECT THE CONTEXT TO MAKE UP THE BACKDROP AGAINST WHICH YOUR LIFE UNFOLDS.

SPLIT SECOND

EVOLUTION, BITCH

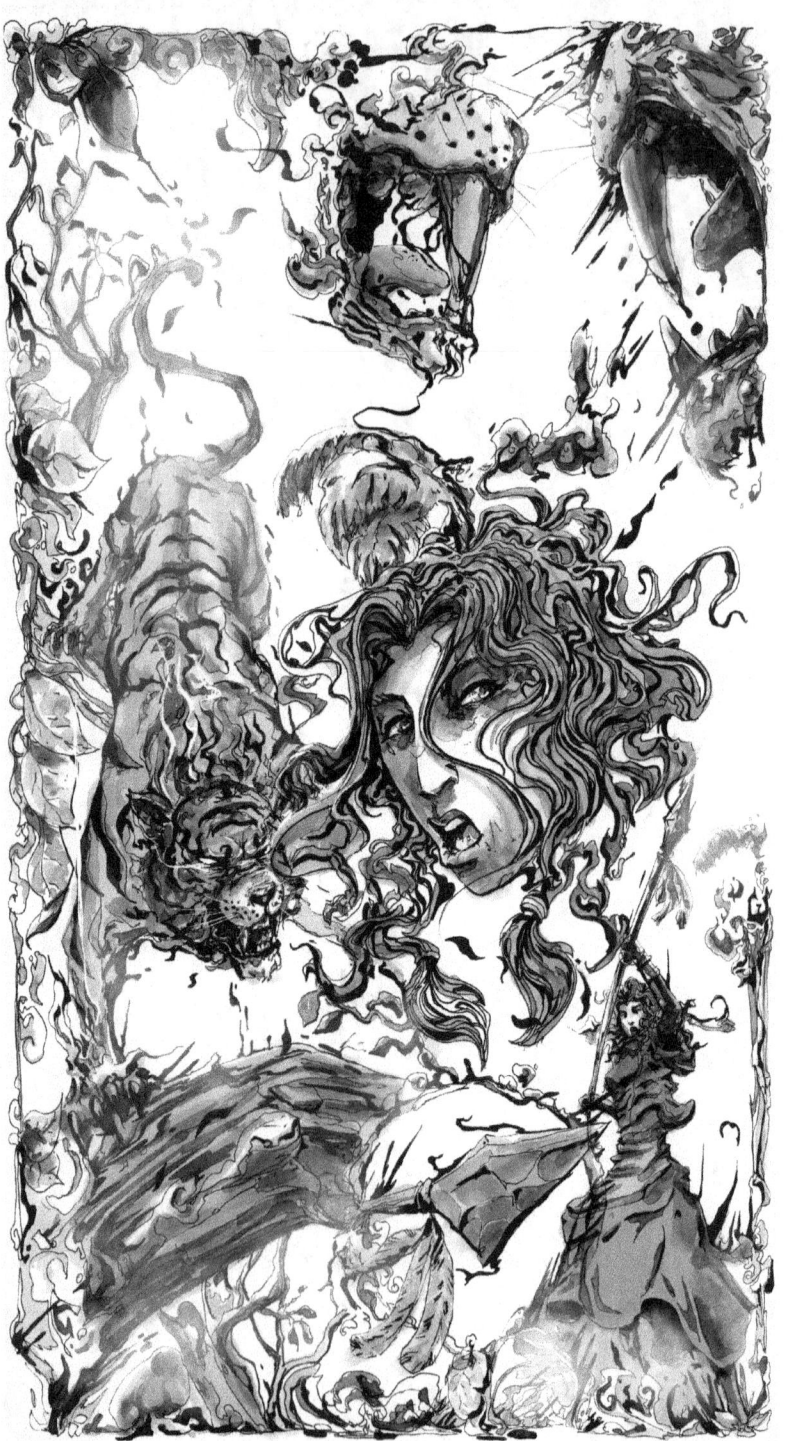

A saber-tooth tiger approaches.

Your ancestor sees it.

What if she spent a few minutes analyzing her perception of the experience?

You wouldn't be here.

You would be a glimmer in the sky if she stopped to think about what the saber-tooth might do to her kids, and whether running to safety is the best idea!

No, in that split second, she grabs her spear and pushes her kids to safety. Adrenaline pumping, her vision narrows as she positions herself between the kids and the saber-tooth tiger, ready for a fight to the death.

YOU ARE BUILT TO INTERPRET YOUR EXPERIENCE AND TAKE ACTION WITHIN A SPLIT SECOND, WHEN NEEDED.

SCANNING...

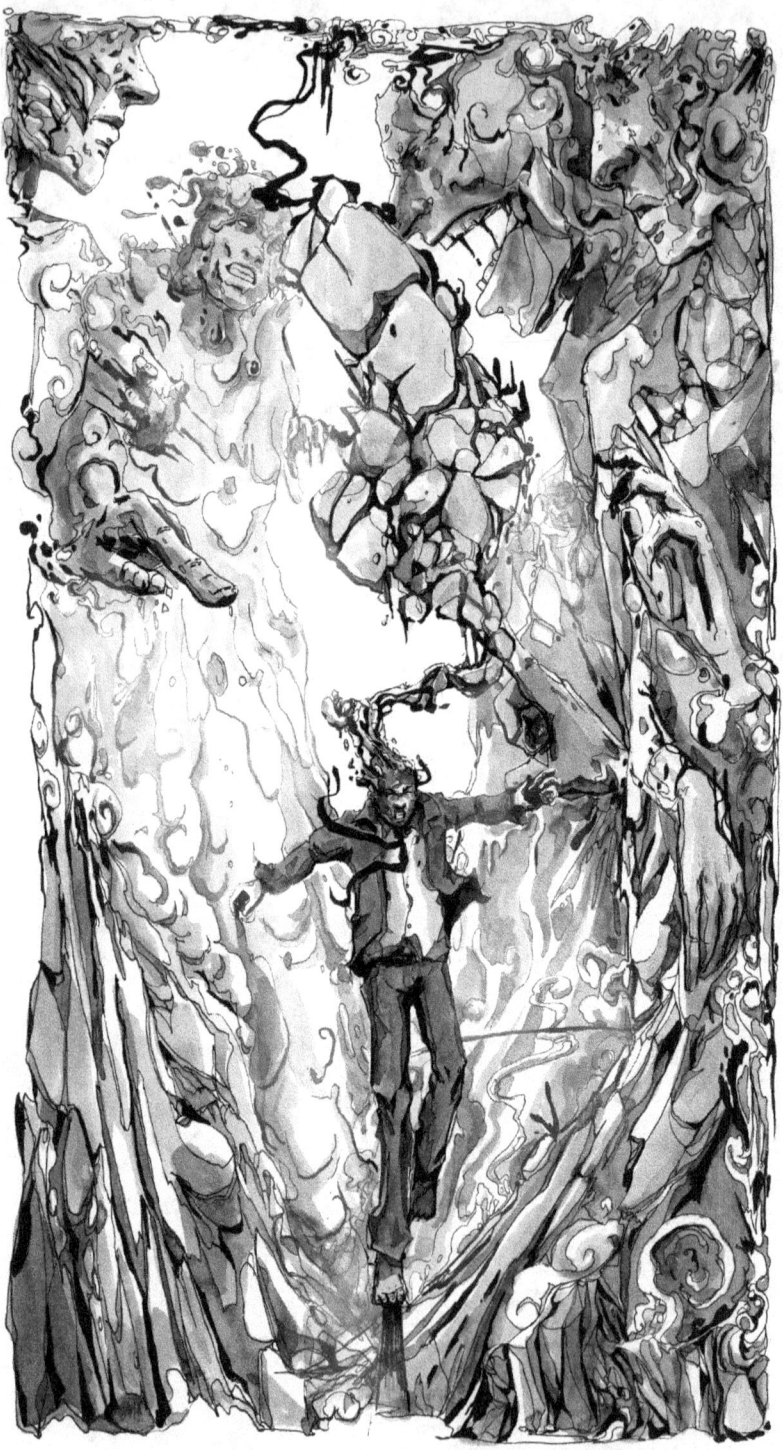

YOUR BRAIN EVOLVED OVER MILLENNIA TO PRIORITIZE SURVIVAL.

It's constantly scanning in the background, looking for threats everywhere.

That's why you perceive words of criticism as an existential threat sometimes. And that's why your body responds as if you're facing off with a sabertooth tiger!

All of a sudden, you become defensive, or maybe aggressive. You're in fight-or-flight as if your very survival is at risk.

As the dust settles, you find yourself at the center of a disaster of misinterpretation and evolutionary response. Instead of a dead tiger, you end up with damaged relationships, a lot to fix, and a shit ton of apologies to make.

MIND THE GAP

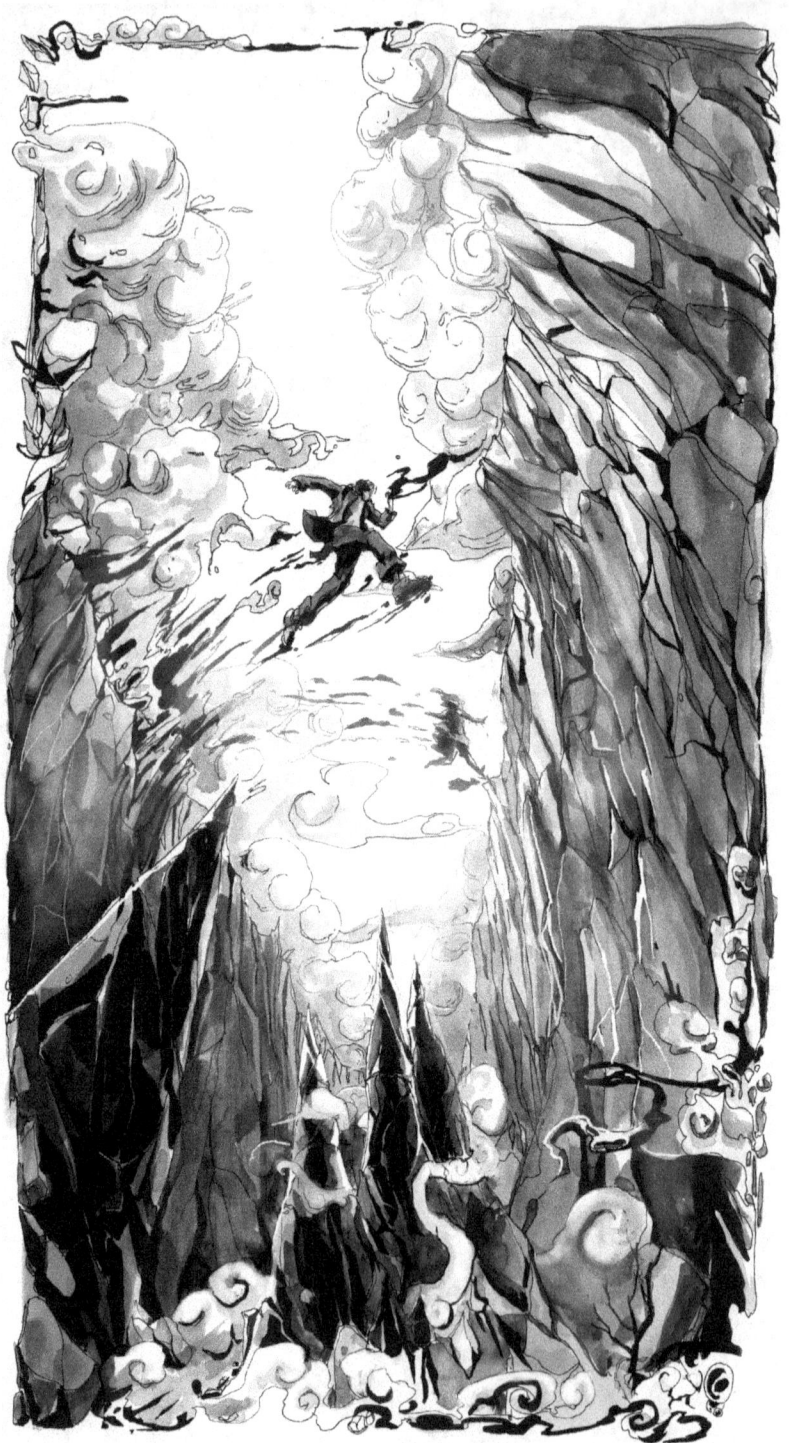

First, things take place in your life.

Then you perceive it.

THERE IS A BIG GAP BETWEEN WHAT REALLY IS, THE WAY YOU PERCEIVE IT, AND HOW IT CHANGES YOUR LIFE EXPERIENCE AS IT'S UNFOLDING.

You are continually making the leap across the gap between what really is and what you want, imagine, perceive, construct, desire, or make it up to be.

By doing so, you unwittingly shape how you think, the words you say, and what you do.

It takes work to mind the gap.

It takes presence to alter your perception.

It takes a lifetime to master your thoughts, words, and actions.

SNAP OUT OF IT

YOUR MIND'S MIND

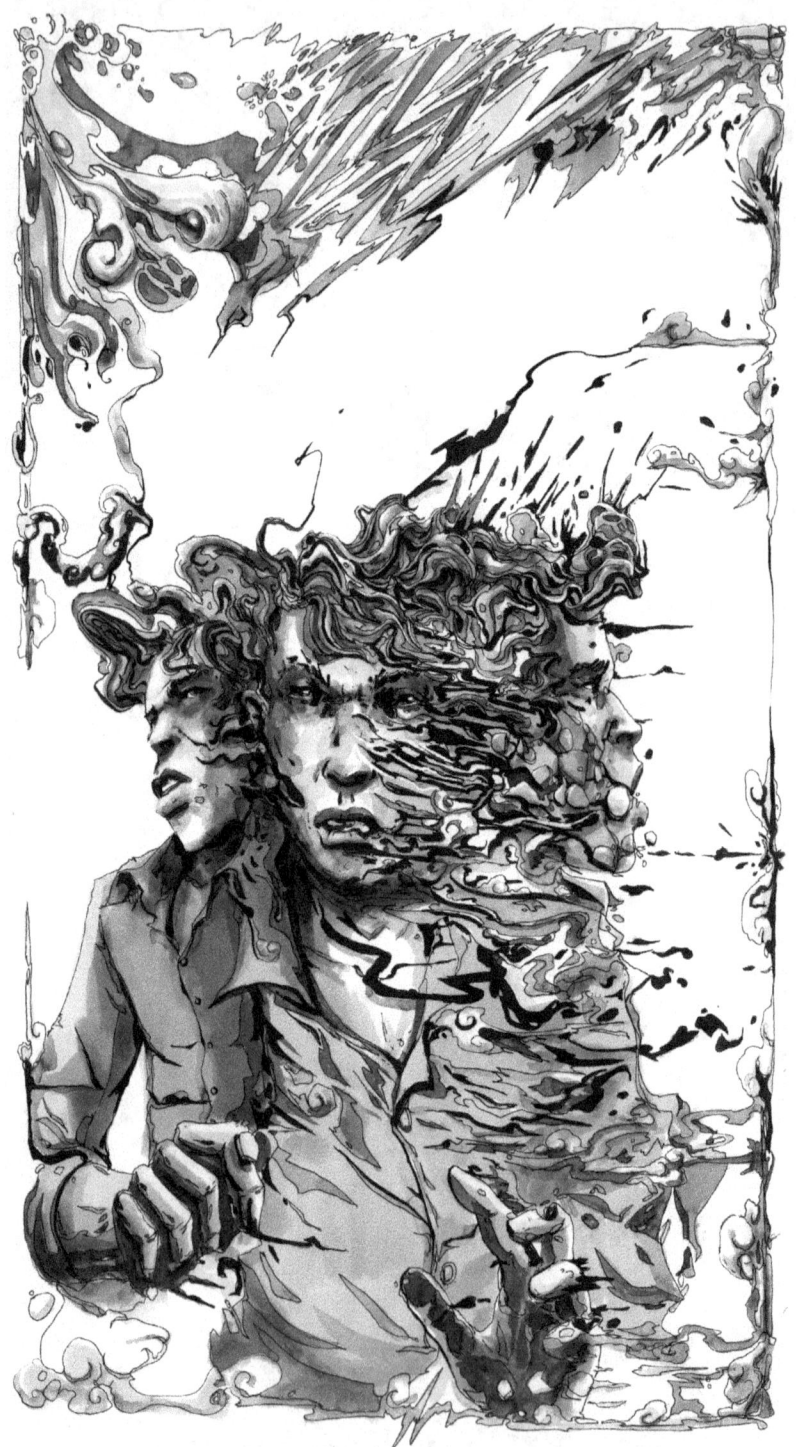

What are you thinking about right now, at this very moment?

Did something just happen?

Are you suddenly reliving a past moment?

Are thoughts racing in your head as you try to make connections, justify, and rationalize?

Maybe you're daydreaming—busy constructing a future vision of the great things you will make happen in the few months or years to come.

Suddenly you snap out of it. A few minutes have passed, maybe more.

THE MOMENT IS GONE.

Your mind has a mind of its own.

Always working nonstop.

Unless you give it something to focus on, it will rip you out of the present moment and teleport you to the past or the future.

The result is you're no longer here, no longer in the moment.

Sometimes you may want to review a past event, see it in a new light, learn from it, or just revel in a feeling of joy you felt before.

At times you may use daydreaming as a powerful way to open up creative possibilities and inspire ideas.

Left unchecked, however, your mind will take you on a ride into the future or lock you in the past, anything to keep you from living in the current moment.

You can't get hurt in the future or the past, only in the present.

The past, no matter how painful, and the future, even when bleak and hopeless, are not real.

FOR YOUR MIND, THE CURRENT MOMENT IS SCARY. IT'S WHERE REALITY UNFOLDS, SHIT HAPPENS, AND YOU MAY HAVE TO DEAL WITH REAL CONSEQUENCES.

MIND YOUR THOUGHTS

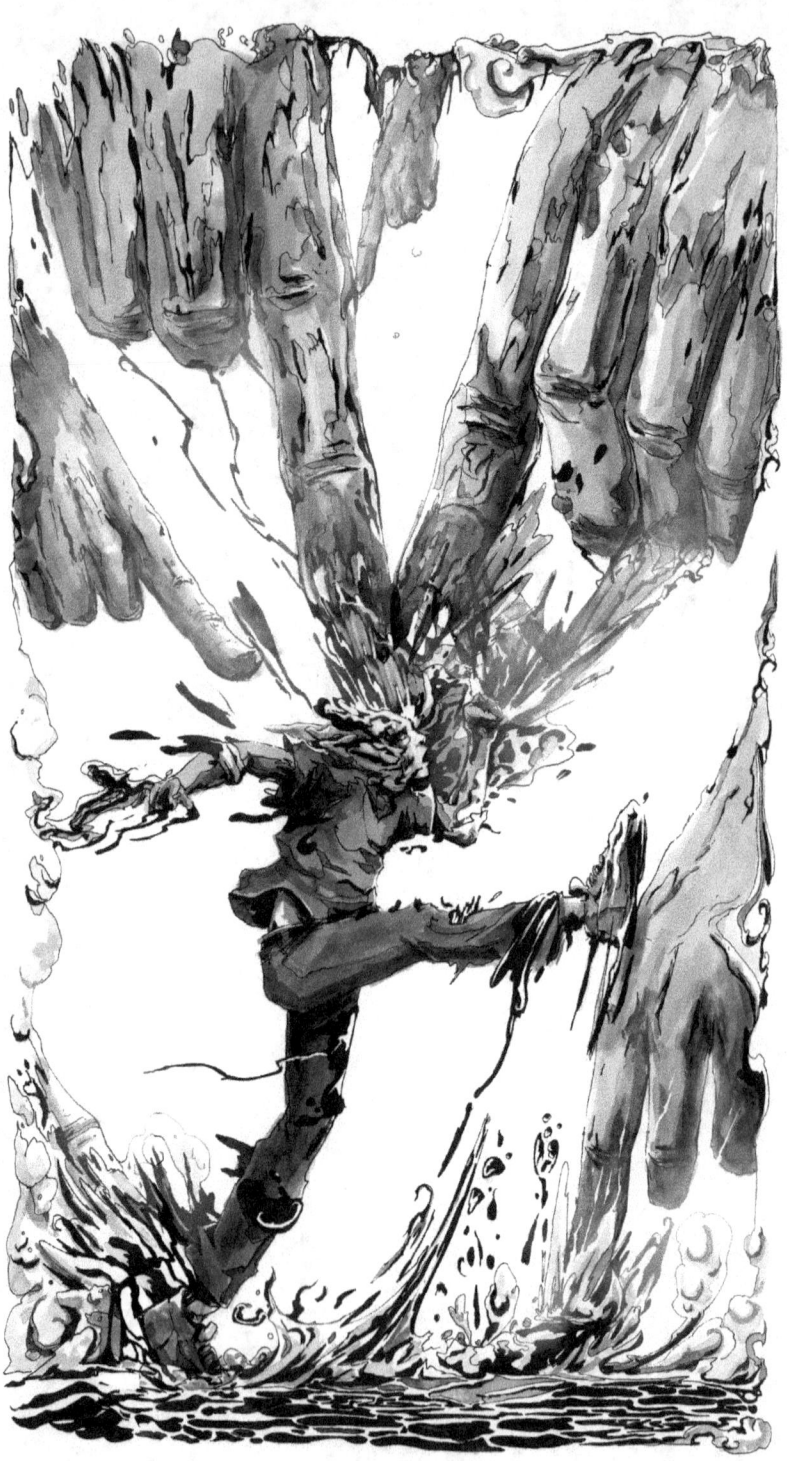

If escaping to the past or present doesn't work, your mind has a million ways to avoid being here, in this moment.

You start your week with a list of essential things to do, new projects to take on, important decisions to make.

YOU ARE ABOUT TO TAKE ACTION, START PLANNING AND GETTING SHIT DONE, BUT YOU STOP FOR A MOMENT TO THINK THINGS THROUGH, "JUST TO MAKE SURE."

You start wondering:

What if I am focusing on the wrong things?

What if I don't get the results I want?

What if I start with regular everyday stuff like email and meetings to get a head start?

What if I find out I don't have what it takes to take on a project this big?

What if I push the hard stuff till tomorrow when I have more time to focus?

What if I don't finish on time?

SUDDENLY YOU ARE STUCK IN YOUR THOUGHTS, AND NOTHING IS GETTING DONE.

RIGHT HERE.
RIGHT NOW.

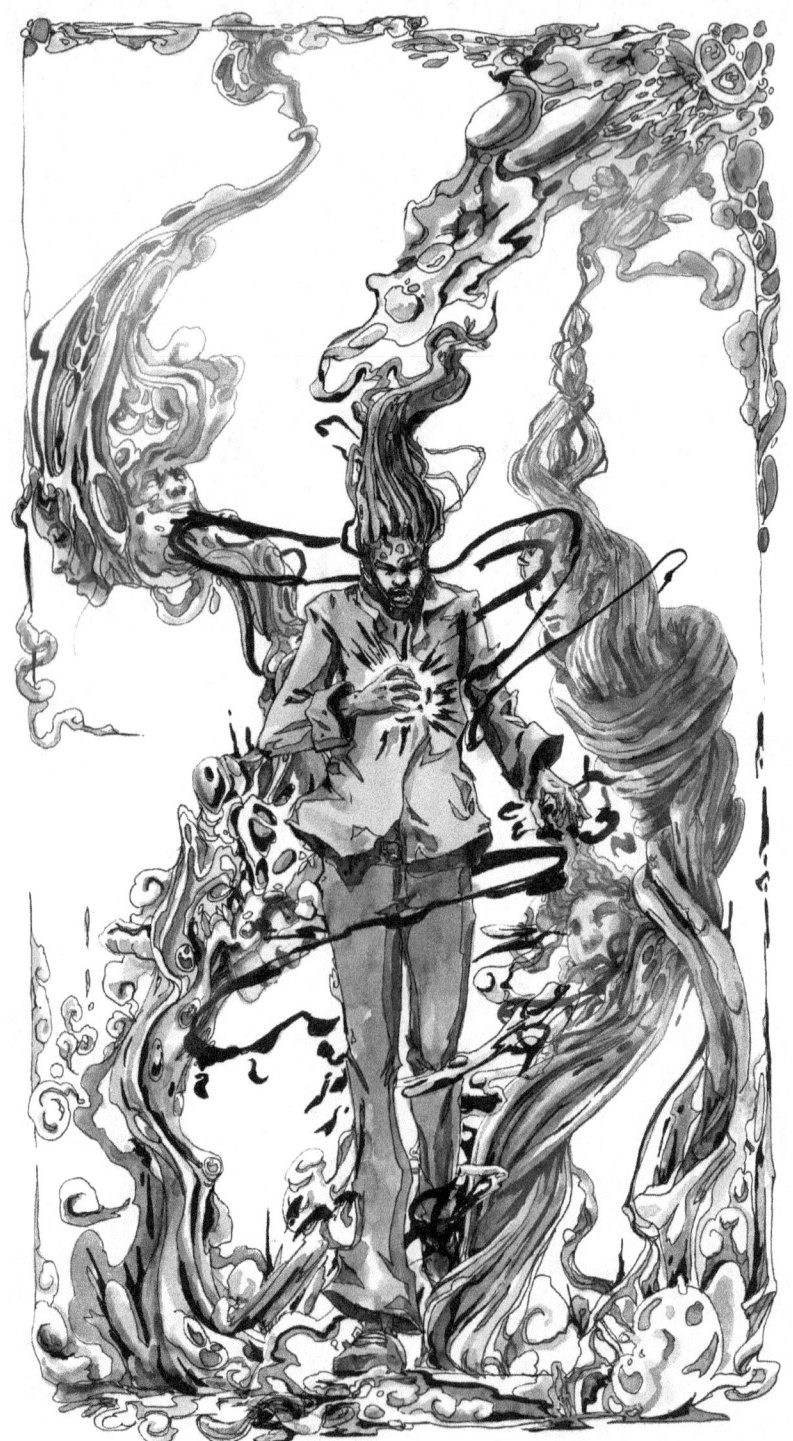

Take a breath.

Let it out.

Take another.

Let it out.

Focus on your breathing.

Feel it going in...and out of your body.

Feel your body.

Feel every sensation in you as you breathe in...and out.

RIGHT HERE IN THIS MOMENT IS WHERE AND WHEN YOU LIVE AND GET THINGS DONE.

Do something.

Do anything to move forward toward the life you wish for yourself.

Go after what's congruent with your words, and what has real impact consistent with your passion and mission.

GO AFTER THE TREASURE OF YOUR FOREFATHERS.

Any life lived in the moment is more fulfilling and more empowering than a perfect life you dream up when you're all in your head.

For some, "living in the moment" has somehow come to mean not caring, releasing your inhibitions, letting down your guard, and just doing whatever.

There's nothing wrong with that if it's your conscious choice.

However, beyond what some people make it out to be, *living in the moment* means being right here, right now.

In the present is where you can take action, enact change, transform things, and make a real difference in your life and the lives of those around you.

GO BIG

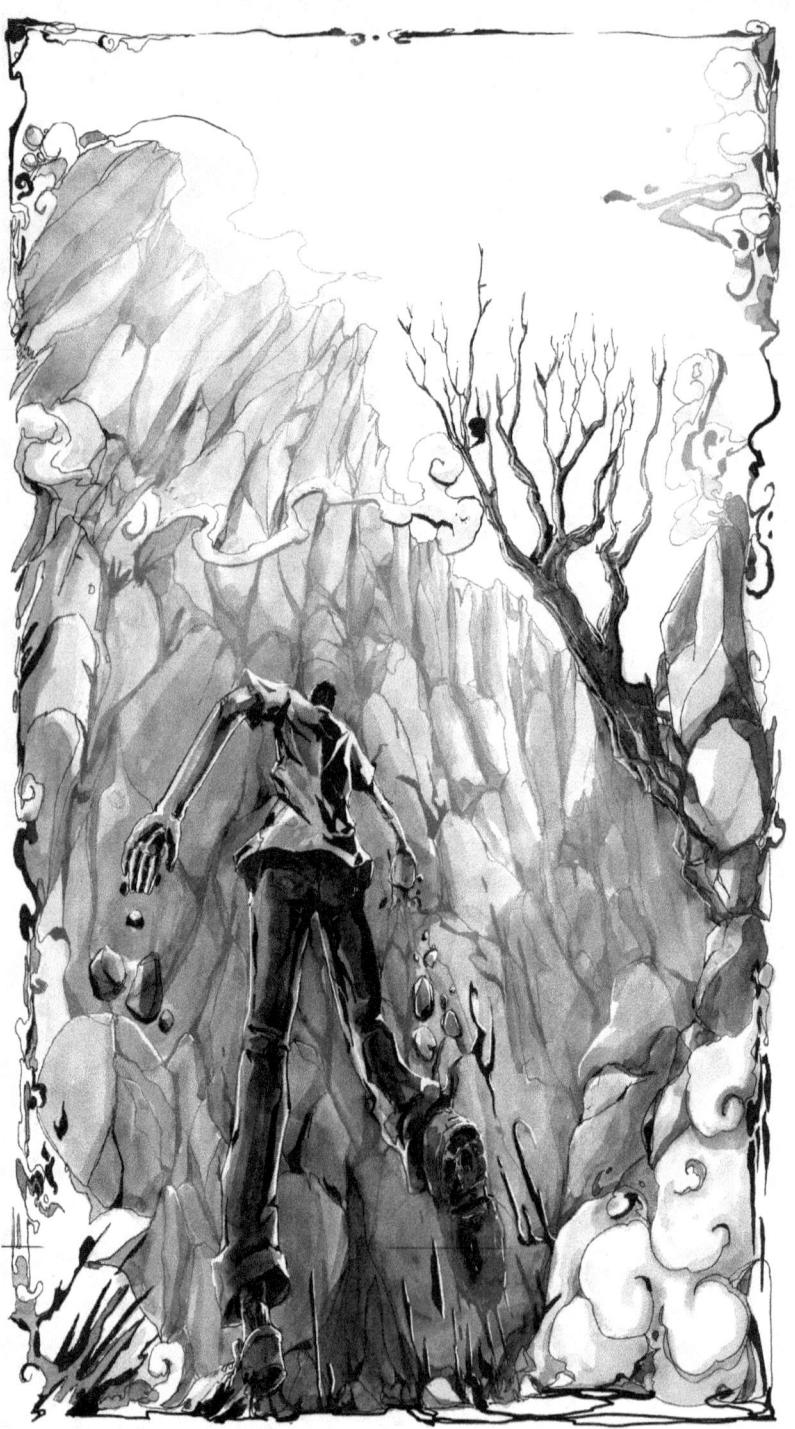

Let's go back to that Wednesday afternoon.

You receive an email invitation from your old boss. One of your tweets is trending. You want to take time to spend with your family, wish to go to the movies, should do your taxes, must meet your work deadlines, and need to attend to a family matter...

Life's demands keep coming at you.

Ideally, you'd address them all, but your time is finite.

SOME DEMANDS REQUIRE AN IN-THE-MOMENT "NO TIME TO THINK" SNAP RESPONSE; OTHERS NEED CONTEMPLATING, PLANNING, AND THOUGHTFUL DECISION-MAKING.

With the pressure mounting to respond, an email from your boss can, at times, seem as urgent and vital as a family emergency.

Completing a project task can fake the temporary satisfaction of spending quality time with your friends.

You clear your inbox and finish that big task. But just as you're about to celebrate, you realize you've put what matters most at the mercy of what matters least.

So much effort, so many hours, and all you have to show for it is the sinking feeling of loss.

YOU'VE MOVED MANY SMALL ROCKS OFF THE ROAD, BUT THE BIG BOULDERS ARE STILL IN THE WAY. YOU'RE GOING NOWHERE!

TEMPORARY JOYS

CHILLED BEER AND A TANTRUM

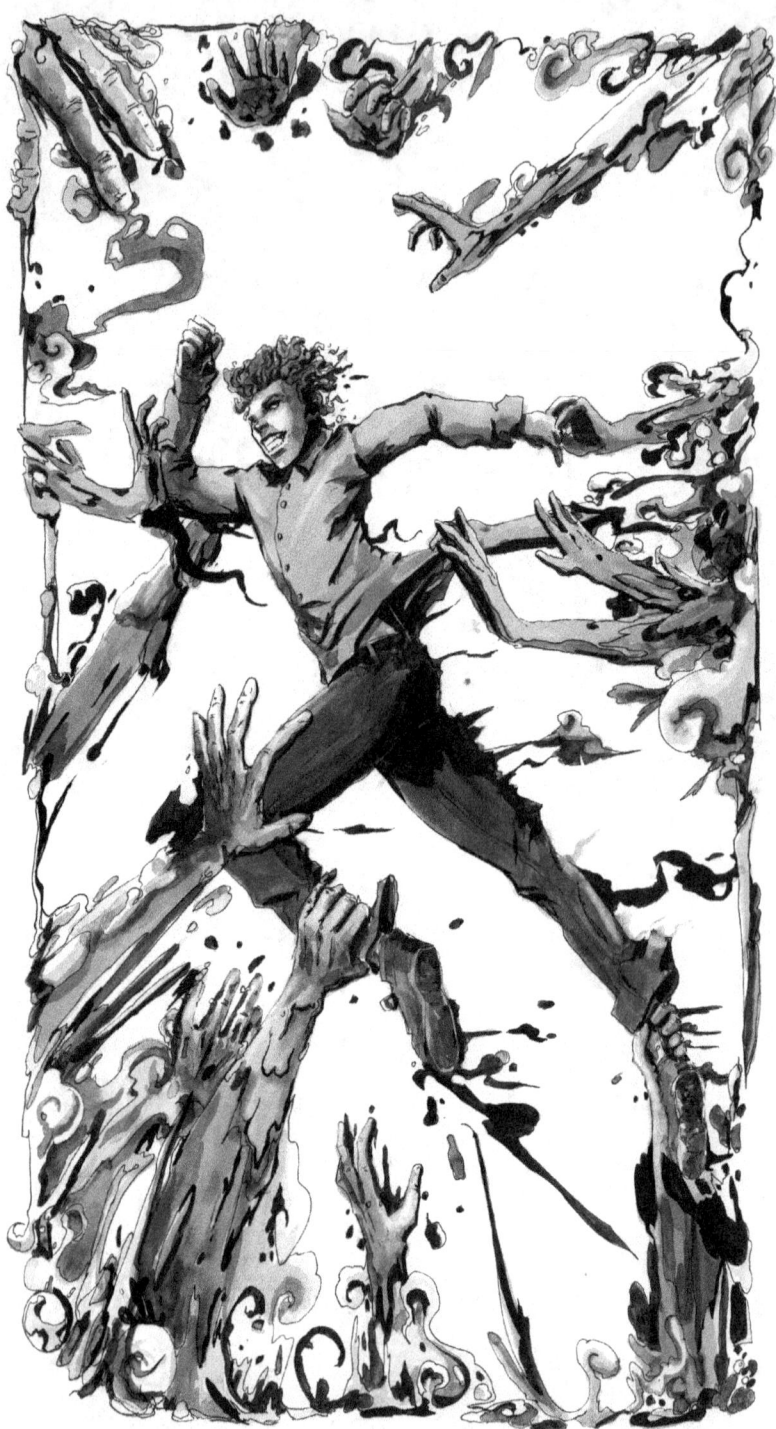

Each life demand requires a different thought process to deal with it.

You congratulate yourself and revel in the joy of clearing your inbox.

But your boss is furious because she's been waiting all day for you to deliver the project plan for her client meeting tomorrow morning!

You take your work home, go all night, and manage to get it to her in the nick of time.

Back home with eyes red and aching body, you grab a chilled beer and sit in your favorite chair.

During your well-deserved moment celebrating saving the day, your daughter bursts into the room and throws a tantrum.

"You promised to play with me, but every time I come, you have work!"

LIFE IS FUCKING COMPLICATED, AND SO ARE HER DEMANDS.

GO HOME

GIVE YOURSELF PERMISSION

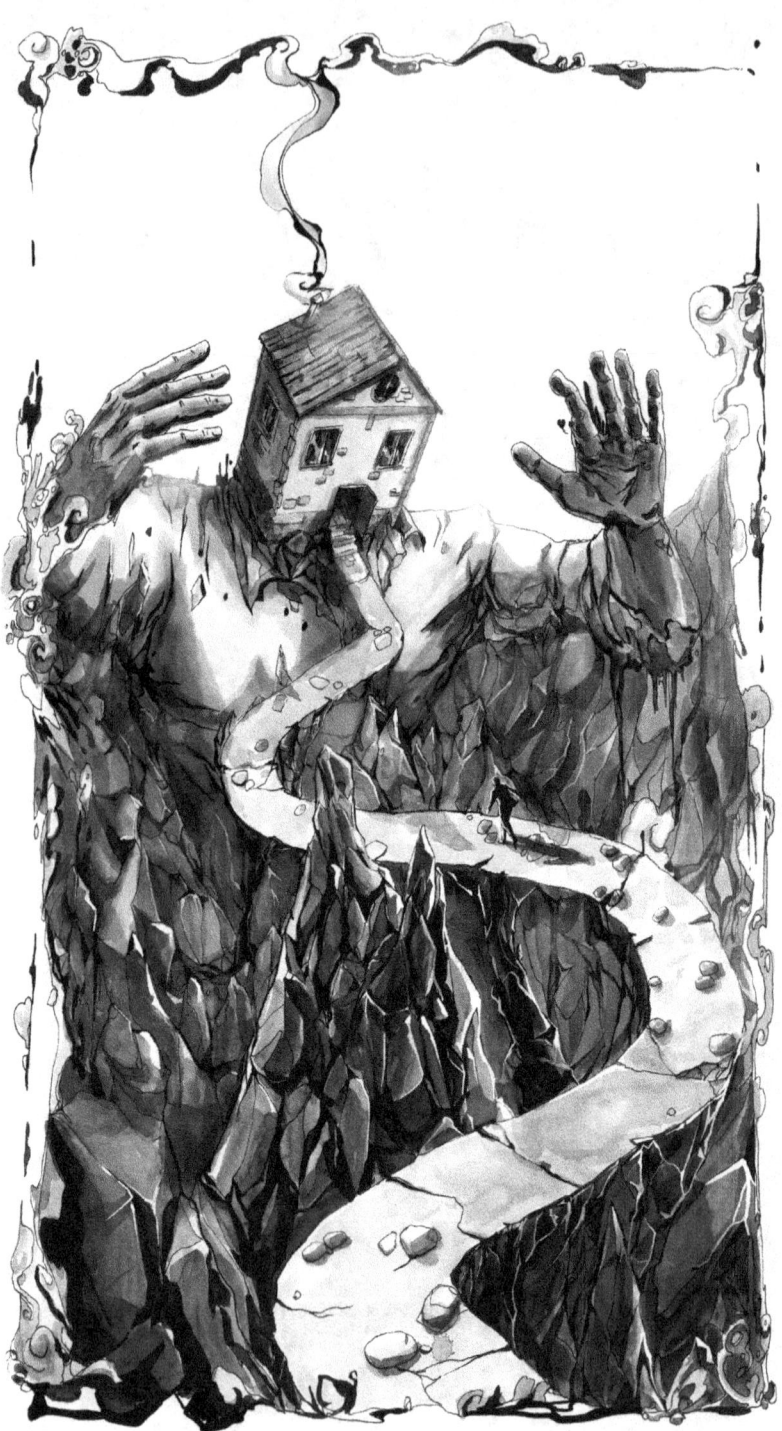

Nothing compares to the feeling of being at home.

Safe, warm, secure, comfortable, and full of energy.

THERE ARE A FEW PEOPLE, THINGS, AND PLACES IN YOUR LIFE THAT GIVE YOU THE FEELING OF BEING AT HOME.

Give yourself permission to seek it.

Go for it.

Make it your guide to the things that matter most, the huge rocks and massive boulders.

Helping a friend when they're in need.

Working on a passion project.

Doing a job that fulfills you.

THE THING ABOUT BEING AT HOME IS, EVEN WHEN IT'S HARD, IT'S EASY. EVEN AS IT CONSUMES YOU, IT FILLS YOU UP. AND EVEN AS IT WEIGHS HEAVY ON YOU, IT GIVES YOU STRENGTH.

THERE'S TIME

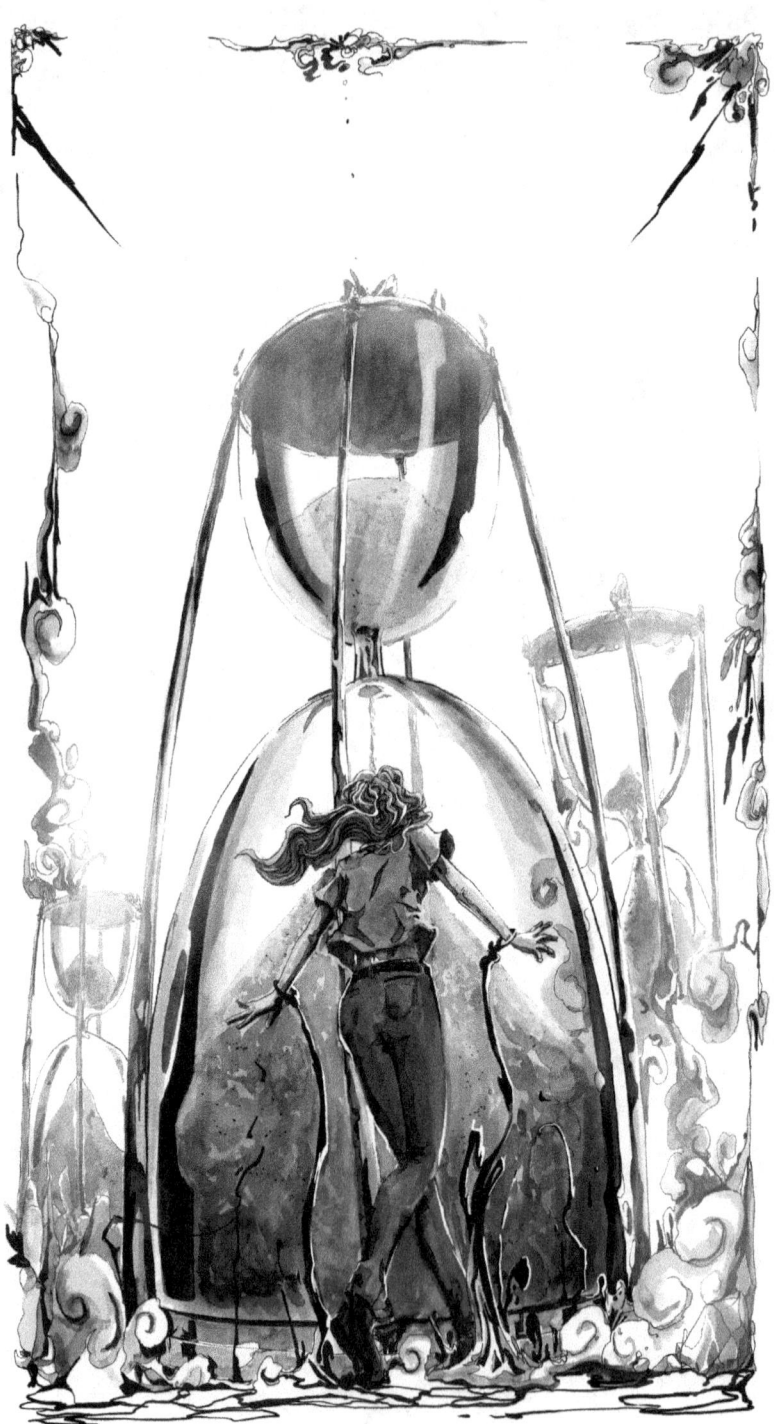

We like to think of time as this abstract constant—that it's the same for everyone.

It's not.

THERE ARE THESE RARE INSTANCES WHEN TIME FEELS ENDLESS WITH NO BEGINNING OR END.

You're in control, moving with poise, eyeing your next destination, choosing it with every step forward.

You feel calm at the heart of the storm life is stirring up around you.

Then there are instances when time feels immovable, standing still.

You feel the whole world is on your shoulders.

You push, and push, and push, but nothing is moving.

It's as if life is conspiring against you, and no matter what you do, you're going nowhere.

And then there are instances when time is fleeting, slipping through your hands as you frantically try to catch up.

Everything feels like it's out of control, your life is unraveling, and the fucking sky is falling.

What the hell is going on?!

Your ship is taking water from everywhere; you're drowning a few hundred meters from the shore, with no lifeboats in sight.

You frantically run around, plugging holes.

You go beyond exhaustion from pumping water out.

But you're out of time!

FUCK!!!!

SOMEDAY

WHO HAS THE TIME?

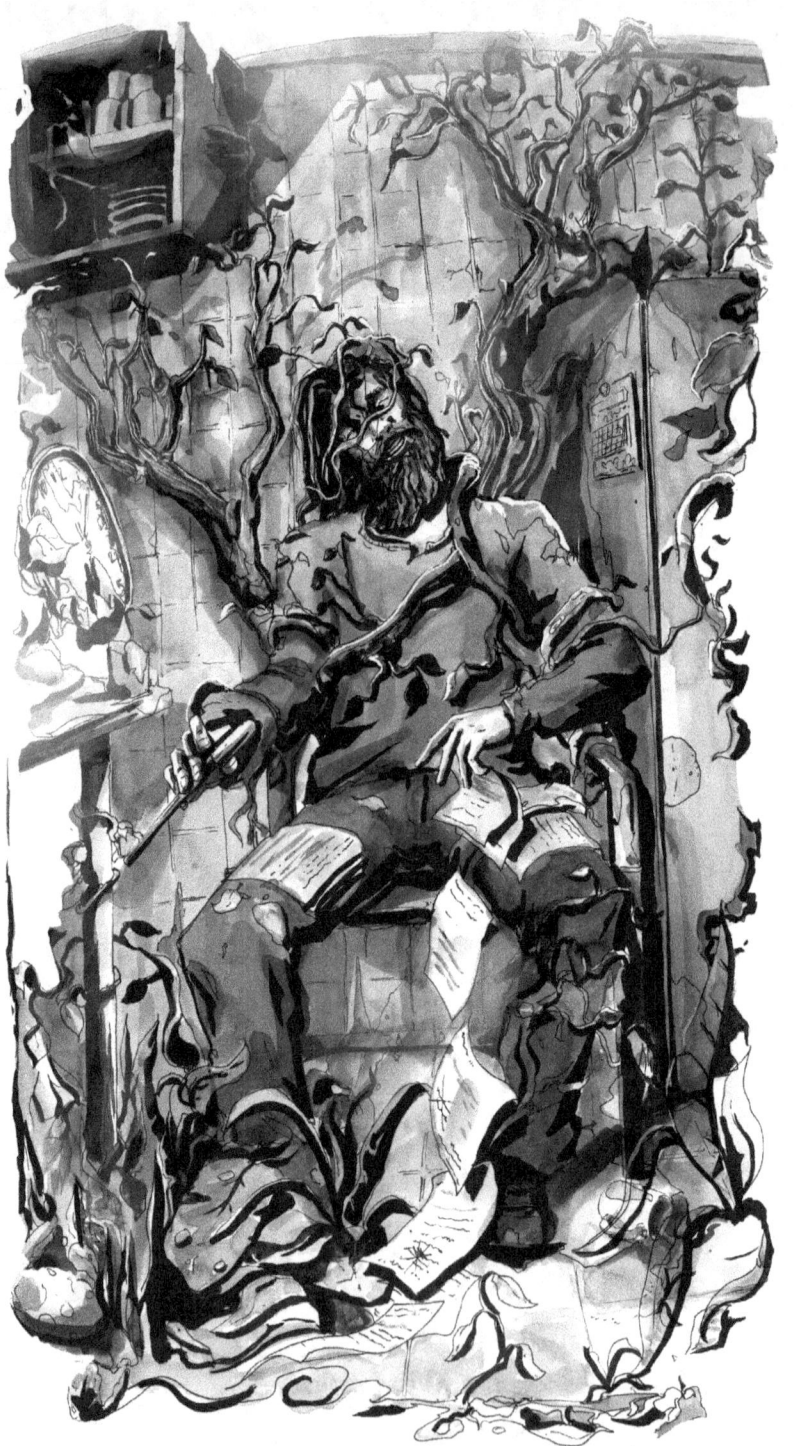

What does it take for you to enjoy this moment you're living right now?

Probably a question you don't ask yourself enough, if at all.

Maybe you don't have time; you're too busy thinking about the future to worry about this moment.

MAYBE THINKING ABOUT THIS MOMENT IS UNCOMFORTABLE. THINGS MAY NOT BE GOING THAT WELL, AND YOUR LIFE IS NOT WHERE YOU WANT IT TO BE.

You tell yourself, *the future will certainly be better*.

It's when everything will be okay.

It's when you'll finally accomplish your life's goals—get rich, meet the love of your life, buy your dream home, and become a valued member of the community.

Who has time to think about the now when there are way too many important things to deal with in the future?!

YOU'VE BEEN TRAINED TO ACCEPT THE "SOMEDAY" DOCTRINE AS GOSPEL.

It started as innocent proclamations by your parents when you were too young to understand, argue, or object.

"Someday, you will become a doctor."

"Someday, you will travel the world."

"Someday, you too will meet someone who will love you unconditionally, and together you will get your own place and build the life you deserve."

Then you go to someday church, also known as school, to deepen your someday thinking.

Almost everything you learn at school is designed so you can someday get into college. Then someday university, work at a big company, go up the corporate ladder—so that someday you can retire and enjoy your life.

Someday sounds wonderful except for the cost—twenty-five to fifty-five years of your life.

But who's counting?!

THE ONE THING

NOTHING ELSE MATTERS

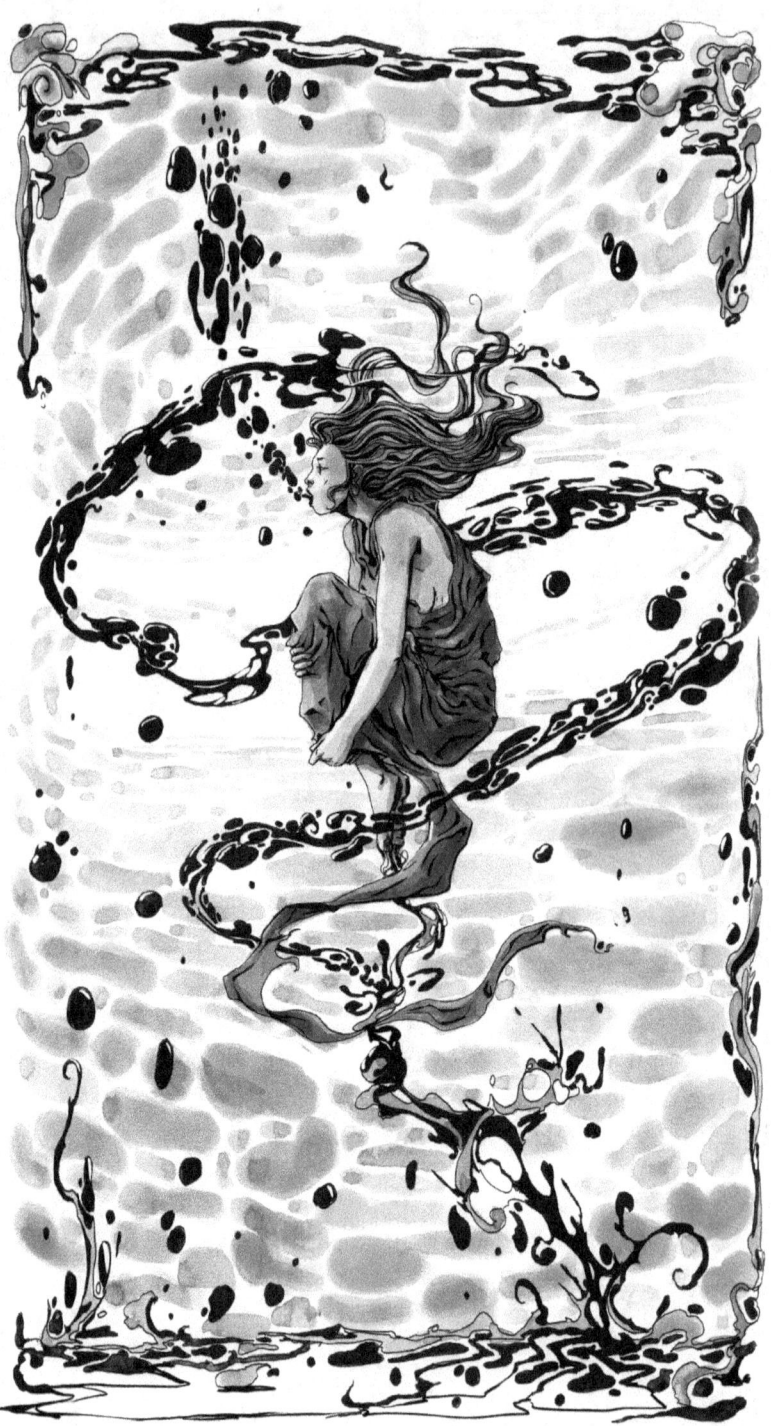

You've probably been conditioned to go through life thinking everything would fall perfectly into place if only <fill in the blank>.

If only you had a better job, a bigger home, a higher salary, more luck, a loving wife, richer parents, a different passport, a successful business, influential friends...etc.

You can never get anything meaningful done with all these "ifs" and "buts" clouding your thinking.

Stop.

Take a breath.

And ask yourself.

WHAT IS THE ONE THING THAT MATTERS MOST TO YOU AT THIS MOMENT?

The one thing that makes a real difference right here, right now.

The one thing that, if lost, nothing else matters.

Stop and ask yourself.

What is it?

YOU MAY HAVE TO PAUSE, THINK HARD, AND GO DEEP INSIDE TO BRING OUT THE ONE THING THAT MATTERS MOST. IT'S LIKELY BURIED UNDER ALL THOSE MEANINGLESS SOMEDAY GOALS.

When you find it, it will be thunderous, loud, clear, and undeniable, making you feel at home.

A FUTURE

TO LIVE NOW

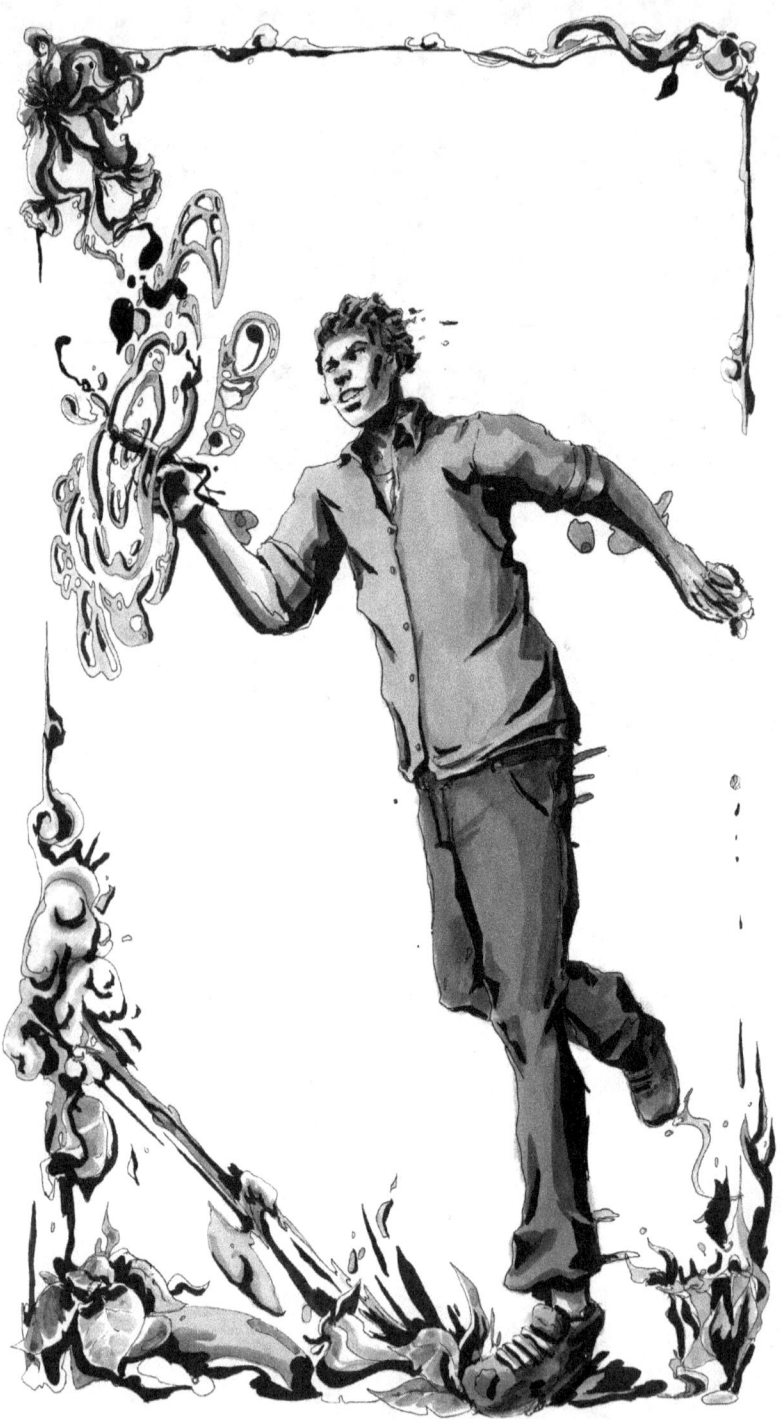

When I asked myself the one thing question, my answer was *"a brilliant, happy, healthy, and loving family."*

It was something I wanted at the moment, in the present.

It wasn't a "someday" when the stars line up and things work themselves out, great things will happen, and I will have my brilliant family.

IT WAS SO POWERFUL IT STOPPED ME IN MY TRACKS. IT WAS AS IF ALL OF MY OTHER FANCY, WELL-WRITTEN GOALS FADED INTO THE BACKGROUND.

This is who I am. This is what gives my life and everything I do meaning.

Its absence is unthinkable.

IT'S WHAT I WANT WITH EVERY SUNRISE, WHAT I WORK FOR WITH EVERYTHING IN ME, WHAT I LIVE AND DIE FOR. PERIOD.

Now, the life I seek finally has meaning, and everything I strive for finally makes perfect sense.

COMPASS

UNLEASH YOUR FULL POTENTIAL

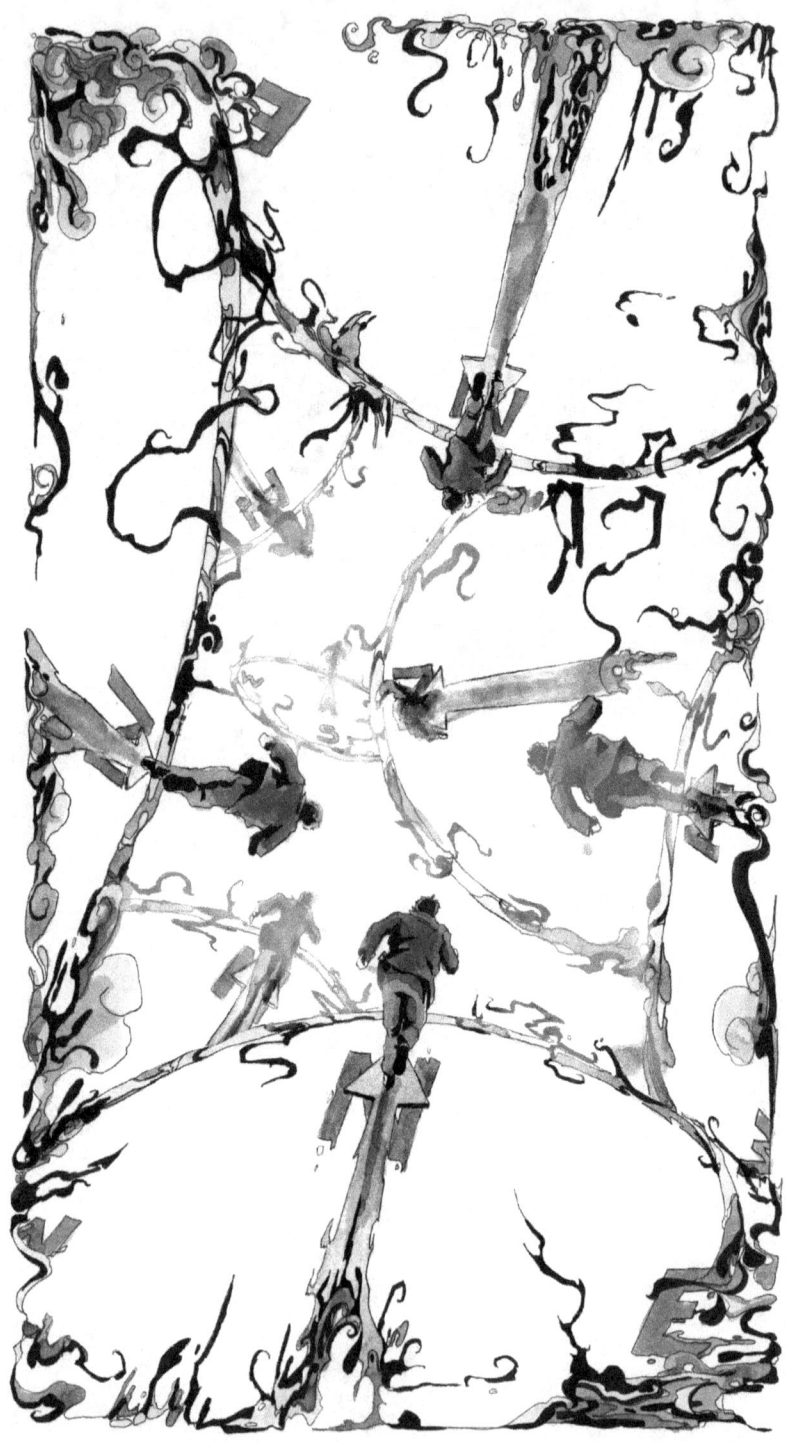

Back at the helm, as the angry waves of the sea of life push your ship in every direction, your destination is hidden.

What do you do?

How do you de-risk the process and make sure you're making the best possible decisions?

HOW DO YOU UNLEASH YOUR FULL POTENTIAL AND LIVE A FEARLESS LIFE OF FEARLESS FOCUS?

You must find your north. It's crucial and incredibly important to reach your destination.

You stop at the port of consideration at the city of contemplation and seek a guru to help you learn.

With eyes open and mind sharp, you bring your all into the process. But you can't help feeling you're not moving. You are learning, but not getting any closer to your destination. As time passes, you get more impatient and frustrated.

Wouldn't it be better to have a compass to tell you where the fuck north is?!

Yes, it would.

A COMPASS WILL HELP YOU NAVIGATE TOWARD YOUR DESTINATION WITH CONFIDENCE.

NORTH

ONE IN A MILLION

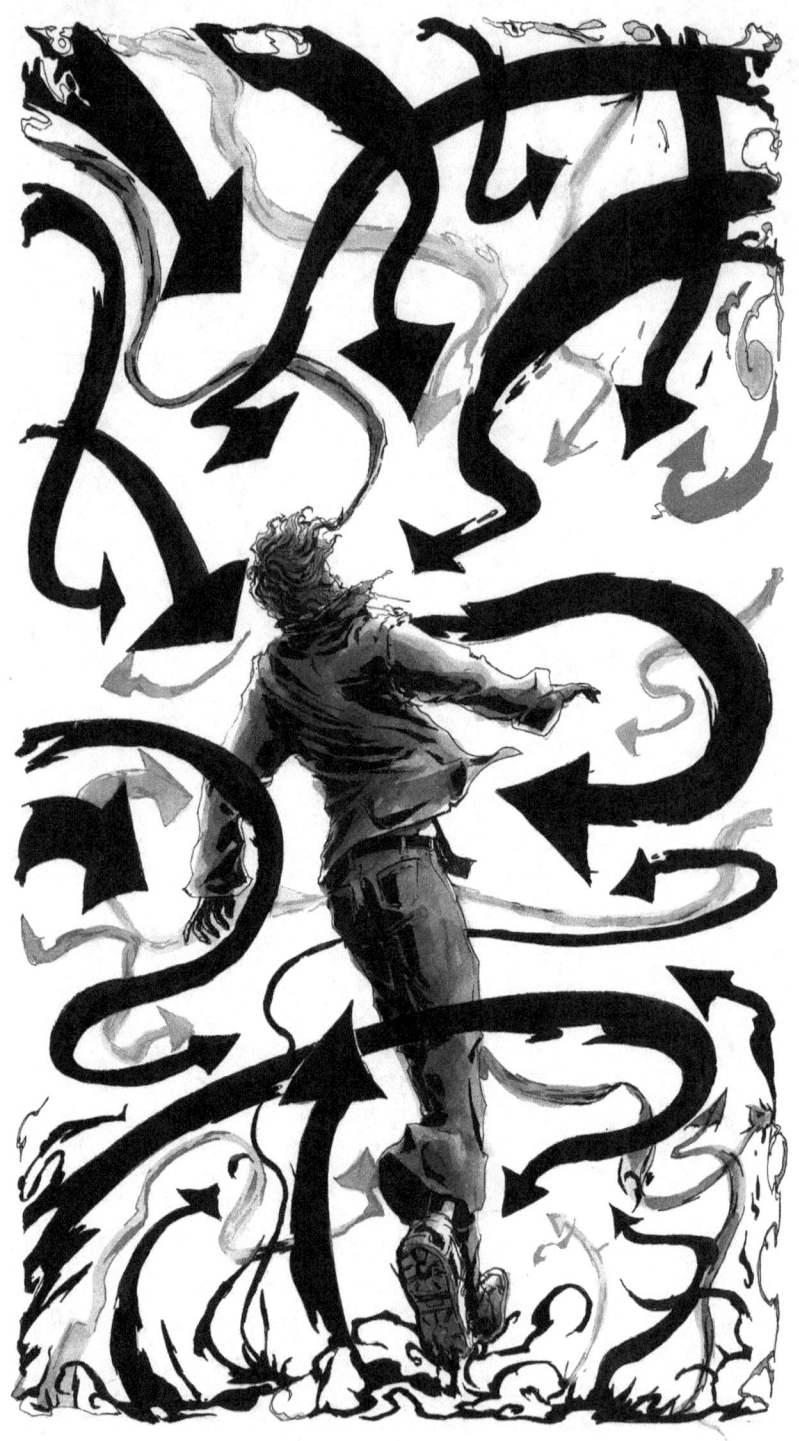

Throughout my adult life, I've been fortunate to come across many opportunities.

Projects, startups, positions, and ideas.

Some piqued my interest, many bored the hell out of me, and a select few ignited inside a fire I couldn't control.

As I progressed through my professional life, the opportunities increased exponentially, and I needed a way to make decisions super fast. I had to see through the trivial and find the monumental.

Whether you have one opportunity or a million, you need a way too.

A compass lines up with the earth's magnetic field; however, your internal compass lines up with what makes you who you are—your north.

It's the fusion of the *people* you love to work with, the future *vision* you're after, and the *legacy* you choose to leave behind. That's your north.

To quickly evaluate any opportunity you have, get to know the people involved, the future vision, and the legacy they plan to leave.

Then check your internal compass and make a decision.

UNLEASH THE POWER OF SNAP DECISIONS BY FINDING YOUR NORTH AND LETTING IT GUIDE YOU TO A LIFE OF CHOICE.

MINDSET

INDECISION PARADOX

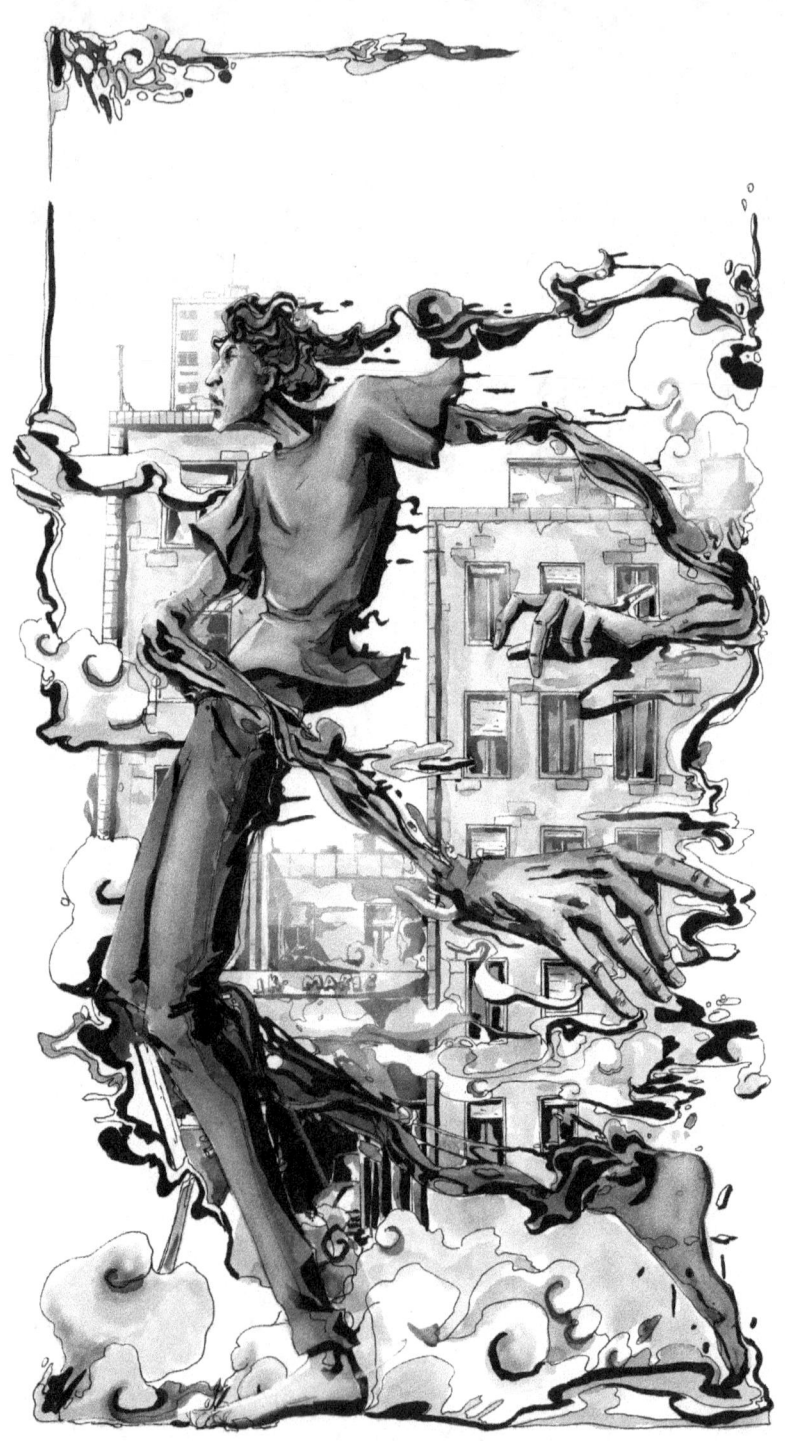

Despite your track record, and even with all the poise, support, and confidence in the world, you still hesitate.

When the sea takes you by surprise.

When all the courage and determination go *poof*.

When things get messy, and your vision becomes blurry.

You hesitate.

Even when you have the skill set.

Even when you have the most complete tool set.

You still fuckin' hesitate!

Even when you have all the information, all the connections, and all the access.

When making simple decisions, you hesitate.

But why?!

Because you think you can postpone a decision. You somehow think you can push it till later. When you are sure. When you are ready. When everything is in place. When the time is right!

Bullshit.

BEYOND THE MOMENTARY RELIEF OF DELAY, NOT MAKING A DECISION IS A DECISION—VERY LIKELY ONE WITH SEVERE CONSEQUENCES.

SLOW IT DOWN

SOMETIMES YOU MUST GO SLOW TO GO FAST

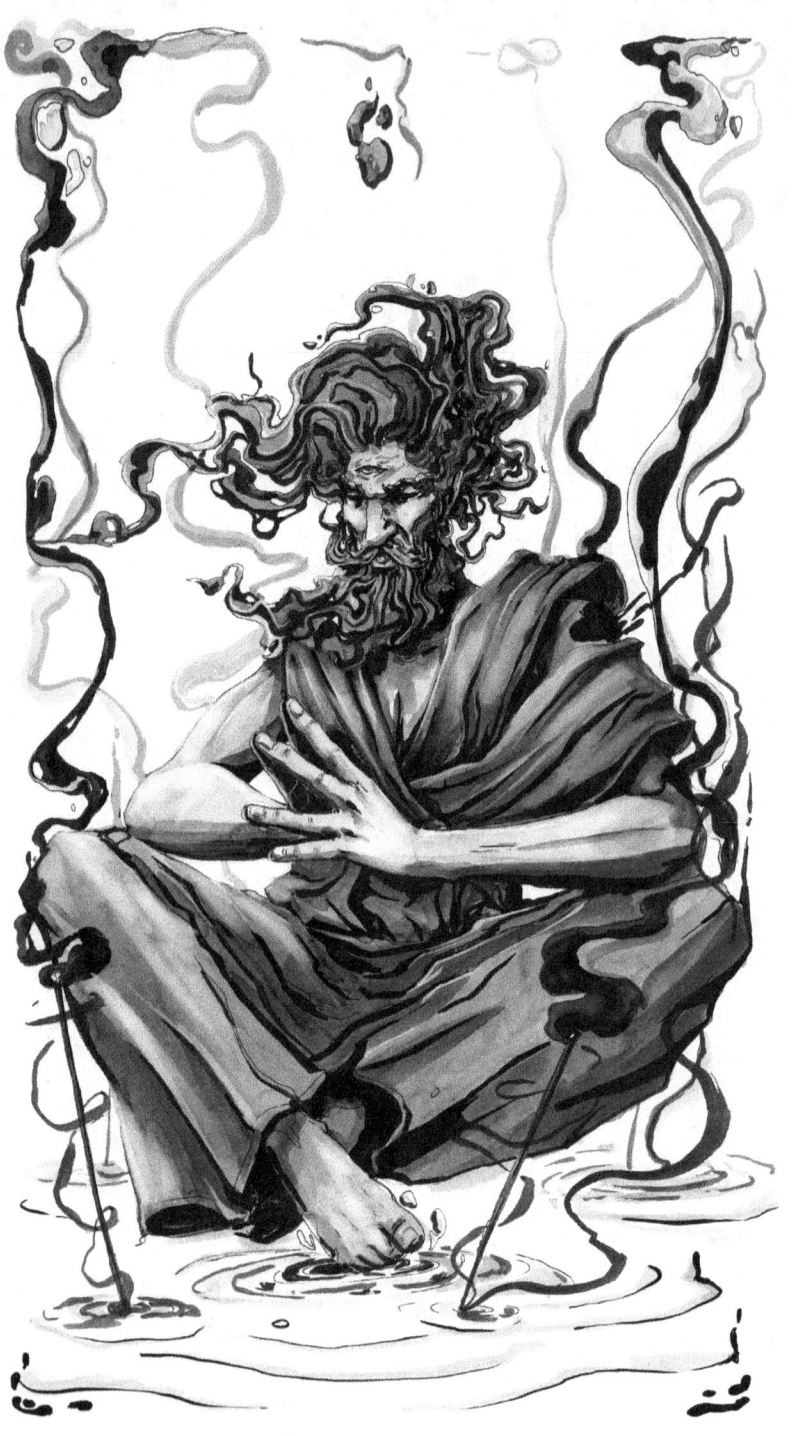

It's Tuesday. Somehow your life seems to be locked in "INSANE" gear, and everything is going a million miles per hour.

The last thing on your mind is slowing down. You need more speed to catch up!

Before you know it, you experience the severe signs of burnout.

Lack of focus, making mistakes, headaches, stress, and uncontrolled outbursts.

Your body, your mind, and everything in you demand you slow down.

How the heck can you slow down, when life around you seems to demand you speed up?!

Let's tackle the obvious first. You are not a machine. Duh!

How you measure your productivity cannot be based solely on how much work you get done.

Instead, you must measure your productivity by your ability to produce better work that significantly impacts your life and the lives of others around you, including your team, company, customers, family, and loved ones.

Slow down to consider what to focus on.

Slow down to make sure it's high-quality work with a significant impact on your life and the lives of those you care about.

SLOW DOWN TO AVOID BEING SWEPT AWAY IN THE CHAOS OF LIFE. WHEN THINGS ARE GOING FAST, AND YOU FEEL A NEED TO CATCH UP, SLOW DOWN, CATCH YOUR BREATH, REFOCUS, THEN GET GOING.

ONLY HUMAN

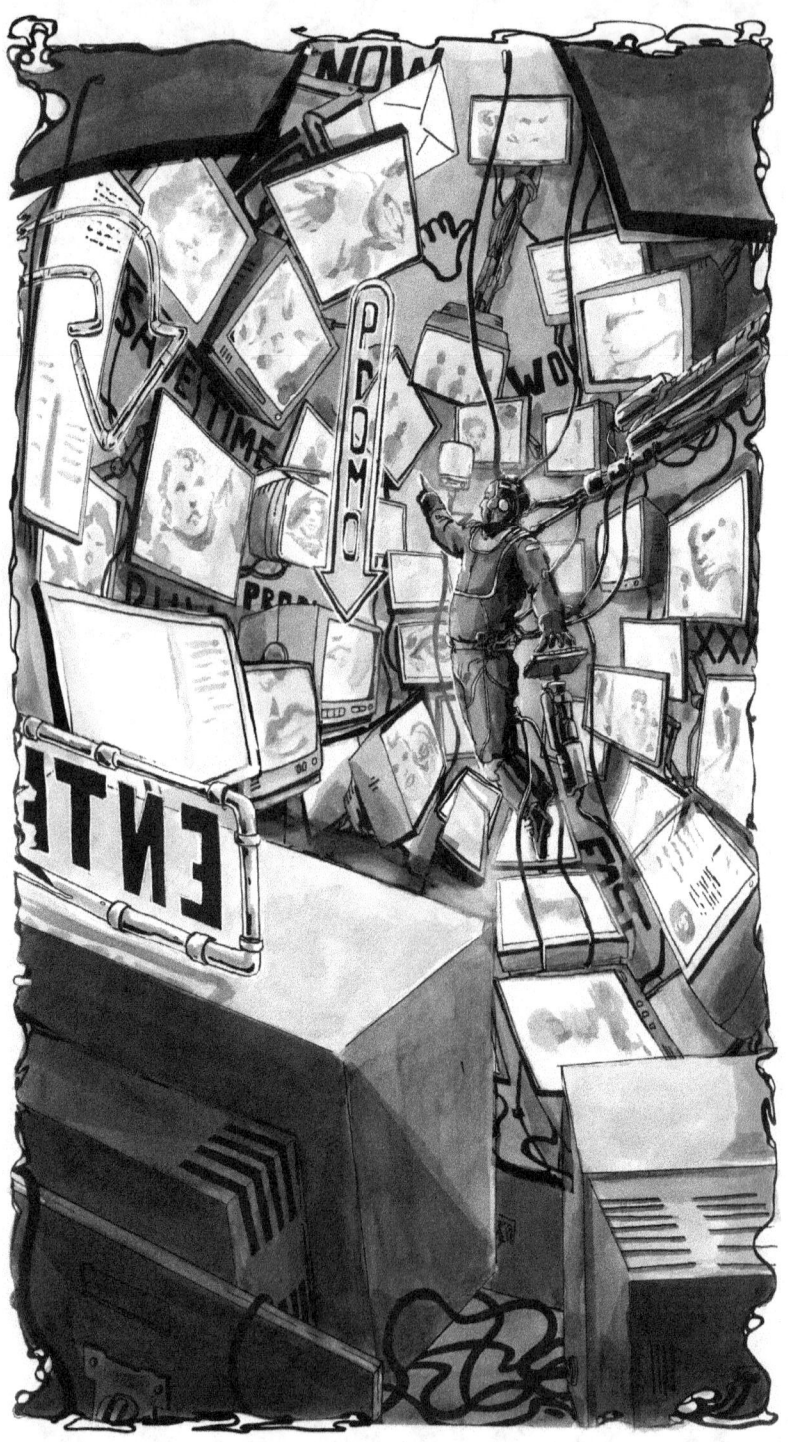

One of our core human traits is adaptability.

But the rate of change, disruption, and tech evolution taking the world by storm is outpacing our ability to adapt at an exponential rate.

ALMOST EVERYONE YOU MEET, NO MATTER HOW CAPABLE OR SMART, WILL COMPLAIN ABOUT BEING OVERWHELMED AND STRUGGLING TO KEEP UP.

Regardless of how much money, influence, or connection you have, you're being pushed way beyond your human limits.

Whether it's the unstoppable stream of emails, the countless meetings, or the ever-expansive list of responsibilities, your life is leaving you feeling like less even as you achieve more.

THE FALL

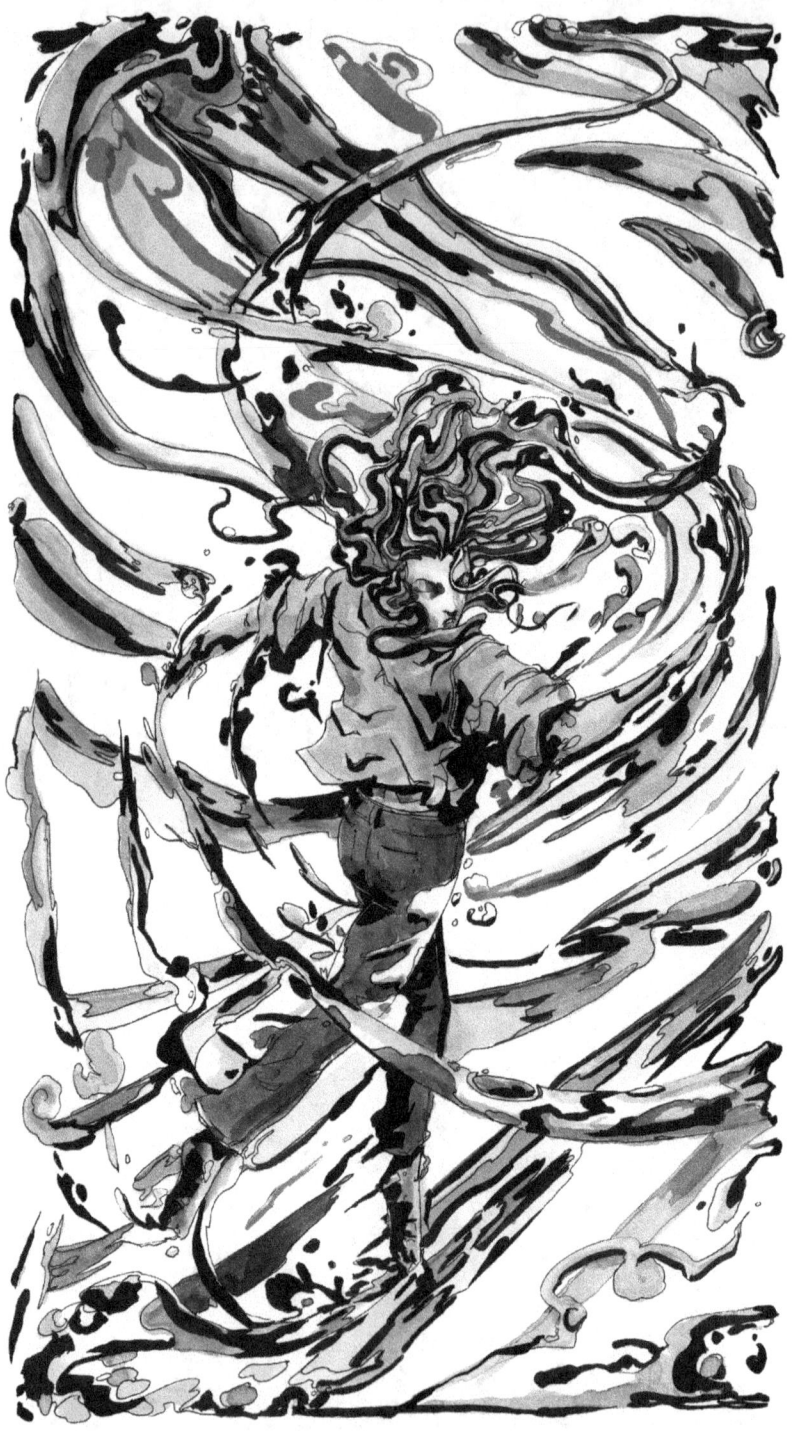

When the pressure is on, and life's demands are knocking down your door, slowing down is counterintuitive. By slowing down, you do the unnatural and go against the demands of the outer world.

But you aim to please, so you choose to keep going, press on, and move forward, even when you need to stop.

You get a boost of energy as you prepare to pull an all-nighter.

You feel a sense of accomplishment when you turn in the project on time.

You fill up with pride when you work through the weekend to clear any unanswered emails or unfinished tasks.

You notice a slight drop in productivity, but you shrug it off.

Things start taking longer to get done; the quality of your work keeps sliding slowly. You notice you're becoming easily distracted, but you shake it off and push forward. You keep getting less done even as you put in more effort.

It's frustrating. You feel like you should stop. Then you look at all of your unanswered emails, and the list of uncompleted tasks.

The thought of disappointing your team and letting down the people who are counting on you is unbearable.

You take five to prepare a large mug of strong coffee, gather your thoughts, muster your energy, get back at it, and work harder than you've ever done before.

After a few days, maybe weeks, you can't remember the last time you had a good restful sleep. You feel like shit. Your body is giving you all kinds of red flags you choose to ignore.

THEN IT HITS YOU.

All of a sudden, your mind is taking eons to process the simplest thought, and your body is refusing to make a move.

You're burnt out and completely drained. Just like being stuck in quicksand, the more you fight, the deeper you sink into complete exhaustion.

SURRENDER

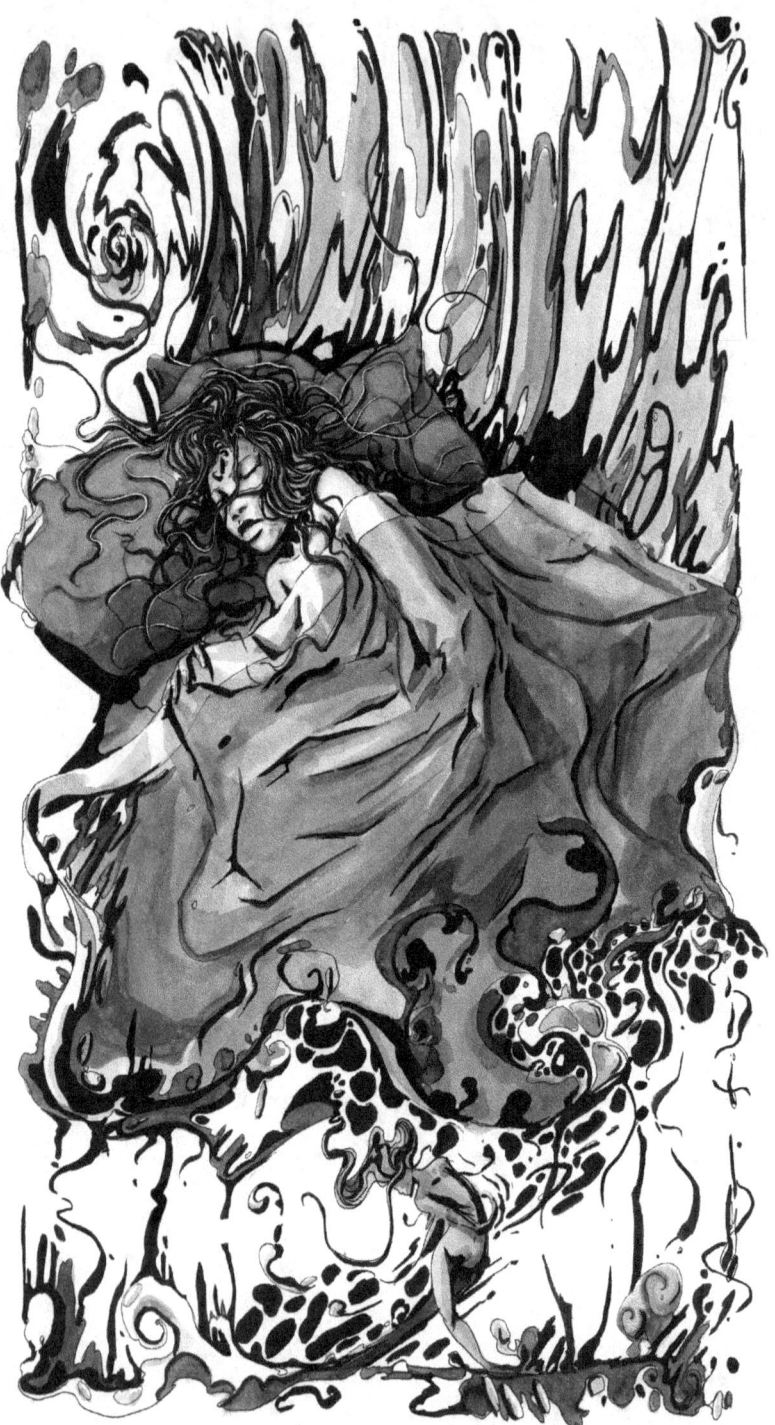

Every minute you spend fighting, every time you deny you're stuck, every attempt to ignore your state and keep going, only pulls you in further.

There is no beating exhaustion, no brute-forcing your way out of this.

You need to surrender. Stop everything you're doing.

REST. LET GO, EMPTY YOUR MIND, RELAX YOUR BODY.

Rest—fully, completely, and unconditionally.

Whatever it takes, no matter how long.

RECOVER

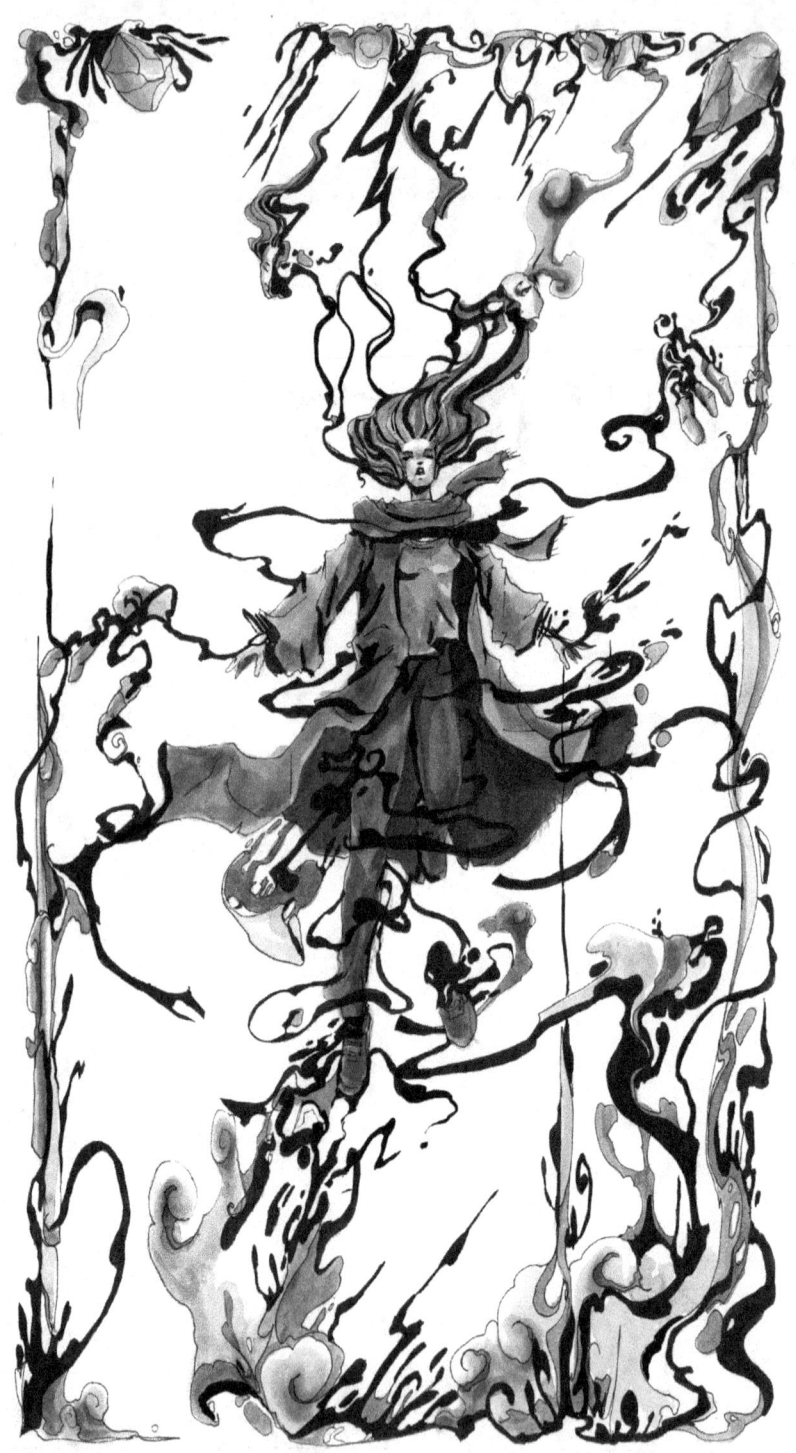

The best measure of your productivity is your energy level.

The better your recovery, the more energy you gain.

WITH MORE ENERGY, YOU BECOME FASTER, MORE FOCUSED, MORE CREATIVE, CAPABLE, AND PRODUCTIVE.

FLOW

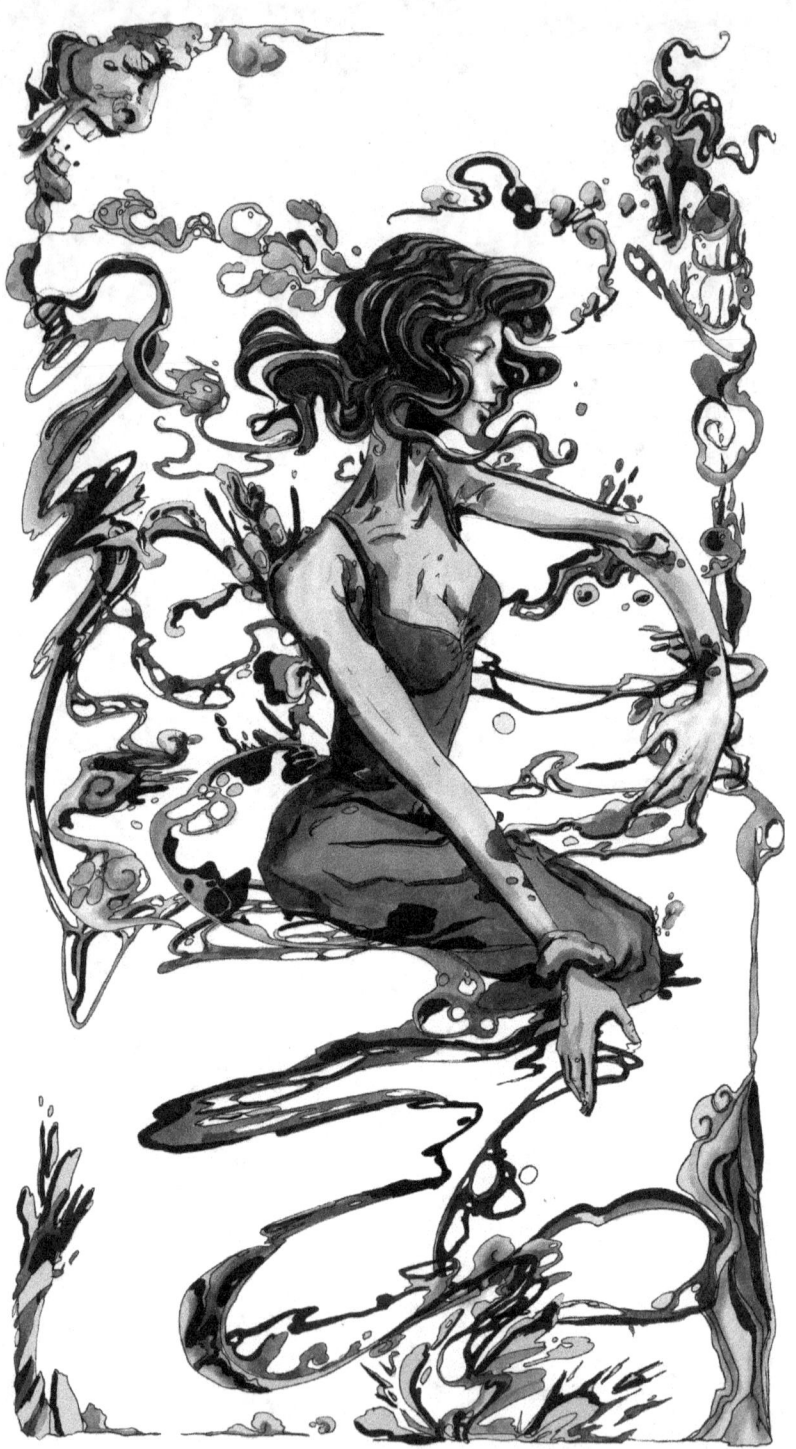

At the highest levels of energy, you operate at a completely different level and produce radically different results; you're almost untouchable.

Things move smoothly, and you get shit done almost at superhuman speed.

YOU ARE IN FLOW; WORK FEELS SO EFFORTLESS YOU MAY EVEN QUESTION WHETHER YOU'RE ACTUALLY WORKING!

At full power, even if things go into utter chaos around you—spinning at insane speeds—you will remain calm and collected at the center of it all.

Clear choices appear, in-the-moment decisions come with ease, and the object of your focus is crystal clear. As you get the most important things done, you feel even more energy flow inside of you.

Fulfilled, thrilled, joyful, focused, and present. The impossible is nothing.

You are your most effective, productive, creative, and capable self.

STEP INTO IT

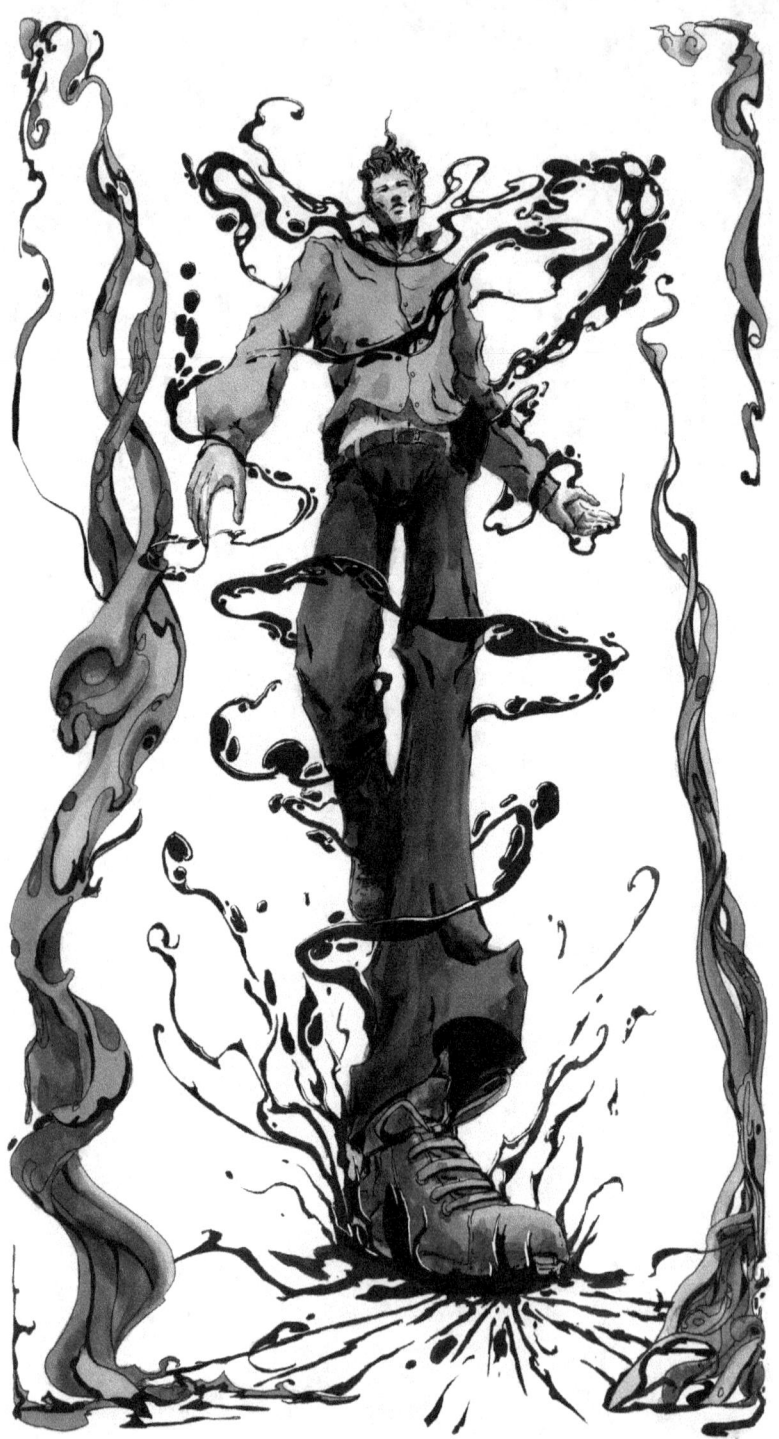

Flow is not a goal, not something to strive toward or to compare your current state to.

You can't work your way to flow.

FLOW IS A FEELING YOU EXPERIENCE, A STATE YOU STEP INTO.

When you choose work that fulfills you, set thrilling goals that get you moving, focus on what brings you joy, and anchor yourself in the present moment, you create the conditions for flow.

80/20

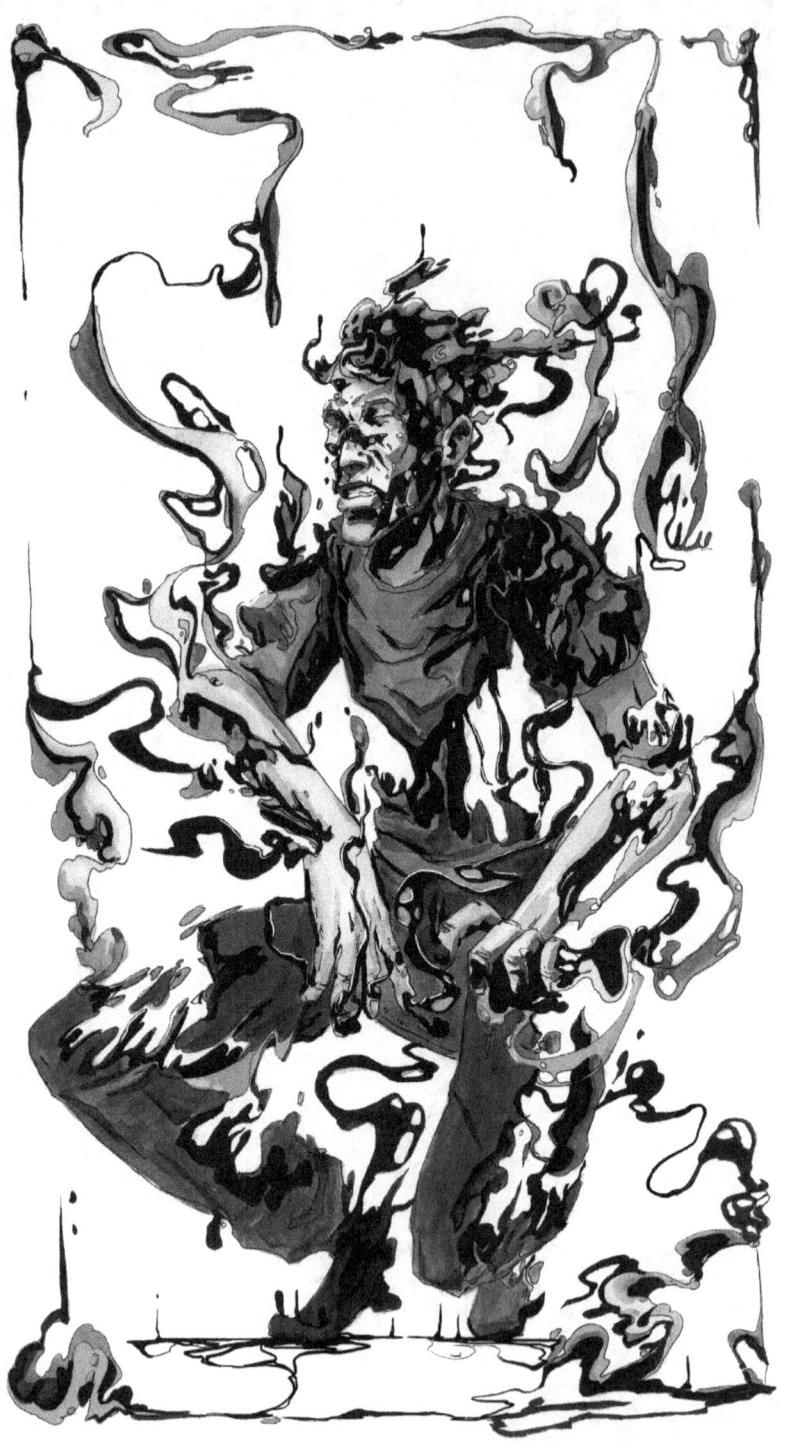

When in flow, you are on a high. You're tempted to use all the energy you've got to move your project forward, complete all your unfinished work, and keep going until your energy is fully used.

Then you remember how the state of complete power depletion makes you feel like shit.

When you are burnt out, you are helpless and powerless as your mind and body give up on you.

It's so much harder and takes so much longer to recover your energy when you use it all.

So how do you maintain a state of flow?

RECHARGE AT 80 AND STOP AT 20.

When your energy is at 80 percent, you may notice small differences in your speed, focus, the quality of your work, and the way you feel.

You just know you are not at your peak state.

If you keep going, it takes more to focus, maintain your speed, and produce quality work.

You quickly use up your energy and find yourself at 20 percent; it's a steep fall to 0 percent from there.

RECHARGE AT 80

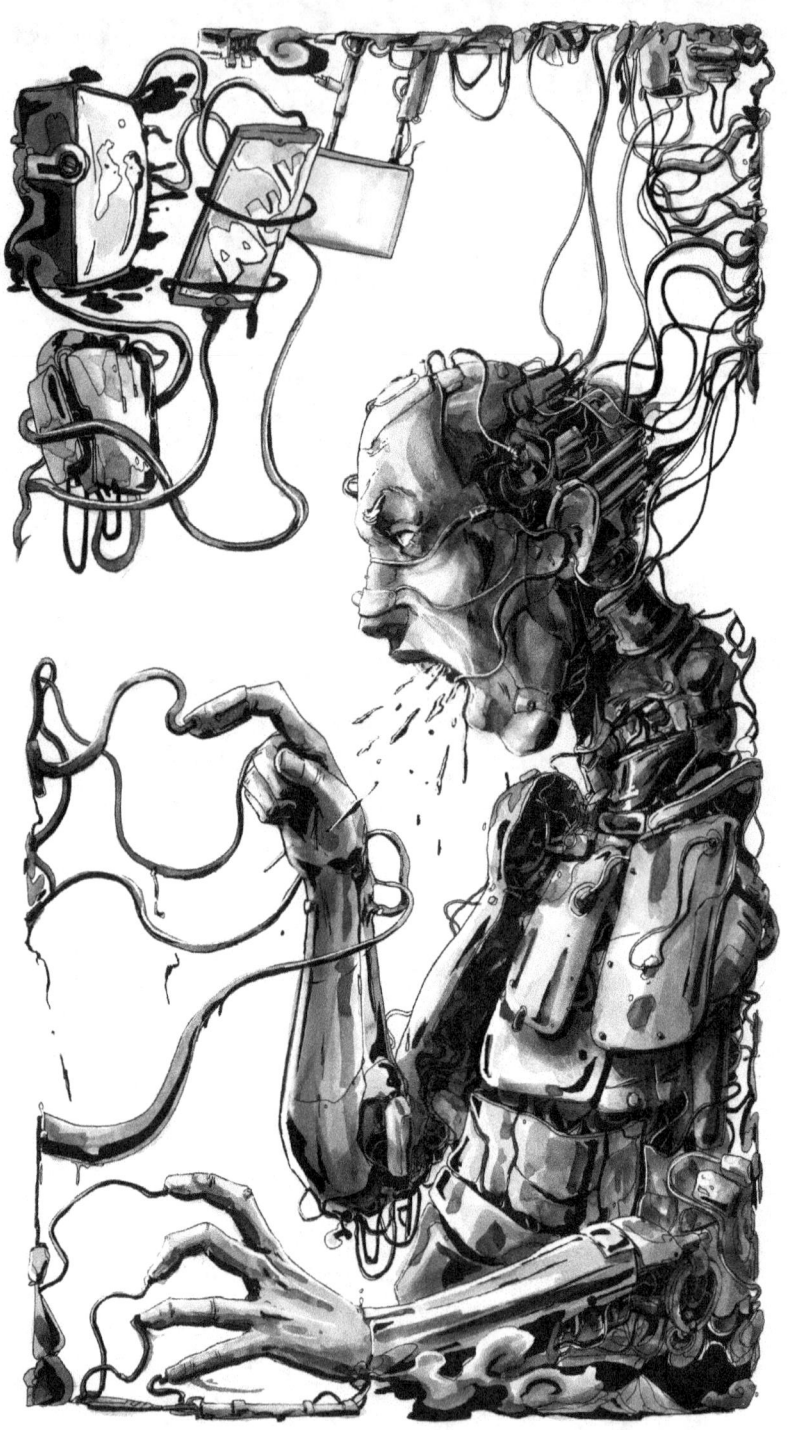

Unless you're battling an angry storm trying to take you away from your chosen destination, recharge.

Unless the one thing that matters most to you is on the line, recharge.

Unless everything you hold dear is at risk, recharge.

YOU MUST STOP AT 80 PERCENT AND TAKE THE TIME TO RECHARGE.

As captain, it's your responsibility to make hard decisions. Only you can decide to rest when everything in you wants to move forward. You must choose to stop even when the destination seems within grasp.

An unforeseen and unexpected rage is always present underneath the calm, so you prepare and save your energy for when you really need it.

Resting, switching off, having fun, or unplugging when you least need it helps you recharge much faster.

There are as many ways to recharge and recover as there are people. And what works at certain times may not at others. So experiment and discover what works best for you, depending on the time and the state you're in.

For me, it's a walk with my favorite music on full blast or listening to a fascinating audiobook.

WALKING IS THE ULTIMATE SWITCH-OFF, AS IT GETS YOUR BODY MOVING AND LETS YOUR MIND DRIFT.

Laughter is always rejuvenating when you feel mentally drained by a hard task or feel that you hit a mental block. Watch a comedy video and laugh.

Watching a really good action movie, for me, is a perfect way to switch off, get absorbed in the story, and forget about real life.

Playing a video game, usually while listening to music or an audiobook, works too.

No-agenda meetings: Taking random meetings with new people opens up new conversations and ideas. Talk about your interests, ideas, books, sports, or music.

WALKING MEETINGS HAVE DOUBLE THE VALUE.

Playing with a pet takes your mind off of work. If you have a dog or work in a dog-friendly office, take one out for a walk and have fun with them at the park.

A twenty-minute power nap can go a long way to giving you energy, as long as you haven't drained your energy. Nothing substitutes a good night's sleep.

Stretch and exercise—a great way to get the energy flowing, and get the endorphins pumping.

Eat. You may be so busy working that you forget to grab a snack or even an apple, so take the time to eat healthy when you need to.

Drink water to maintain your energy levels.

I find it better to get water many times rather than having a big water bottle next to me. It forces me to take a few minutes off. I may even run into someone at the water cooler and have an interesting, uplifting conversation.

Talk to the people most important in your life. A friend, a family member, or a loved one.

Even if only for a few minutes, connecting to someone you care about, listening to them, and talking from the heart may fill you up in a way work simply doesn't.

Experiment with a diverse set of activities for varied lengths to discover which ones fill you up, engage you the most, activate your mind, and leave you ready to step back into flow.

SAY NO

YOU'RE A PEOPLE PLEASER

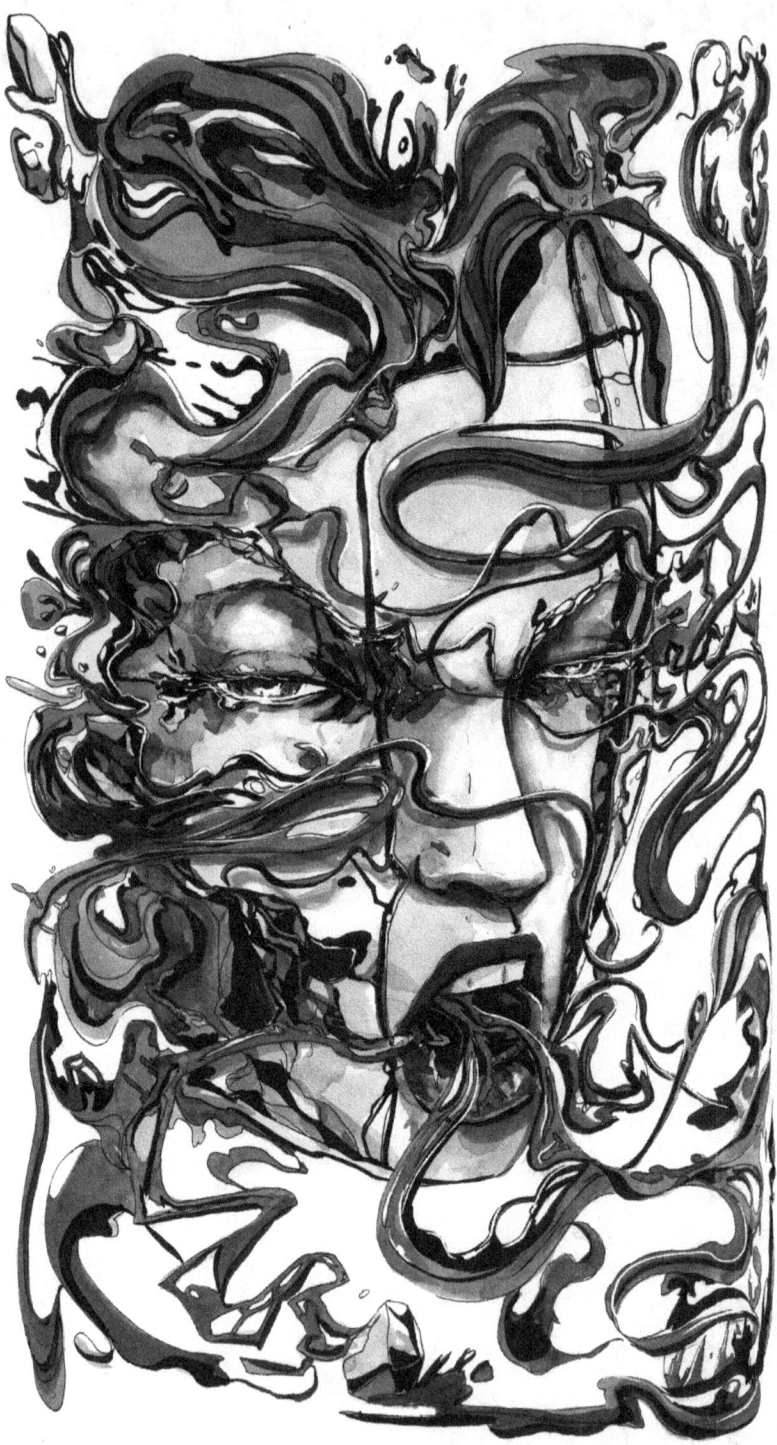

Growing up, you may have gotten some things by throwing tantrums, but you learned very early on to be agreeable, pleasant, and to say yes because when people are happy they shower you with kisses, compliments, and adoration.

Then you discovered "no."

So potent. So powerful.

The first few times you used it, people admired you, laughed, and cheered.

As soon as you started using it strategically, exerting its power to get what you want, the laughs quickly disappeared, and you were met with anger and disappointment.

During your formative years, family is your world, you have no grasp of how vast the actual world is. To you, family is the source of sustenance, protection, and emotional fulfillment.

In the absence of any other challenger, their authority is almost absolute. Saying no to them starts with discovery swiftly followed by prohibition.

They are the only ones qualified and capable of using "no" and wielding its power. You're a child who's supposed to listen to your parents.

Your parents know what's best, and when you challenge them, you put yourself at risk because you're still too young.

Simply put, you were never trained to use "no." Therefore, you have no idea just how powerful it is.

YOU MAY NOT EVEN REALIZE YOU ARE SO AFRAID OF SAYING NO THAT YOU OFTEN SAY YES WHEN YOU WANT TO SAY NO!

You take on calls you should've ignored.

You take on projects out of your scope.

You agree to impossible deadlines because the CEO asked.

You stay on telemarketing calls because you do not want to be rude to someone you don't know who's invading your privacy!

Yeah, you say yes a lot when you should say no. No. NO. NO NO NO.

NO IS A YES

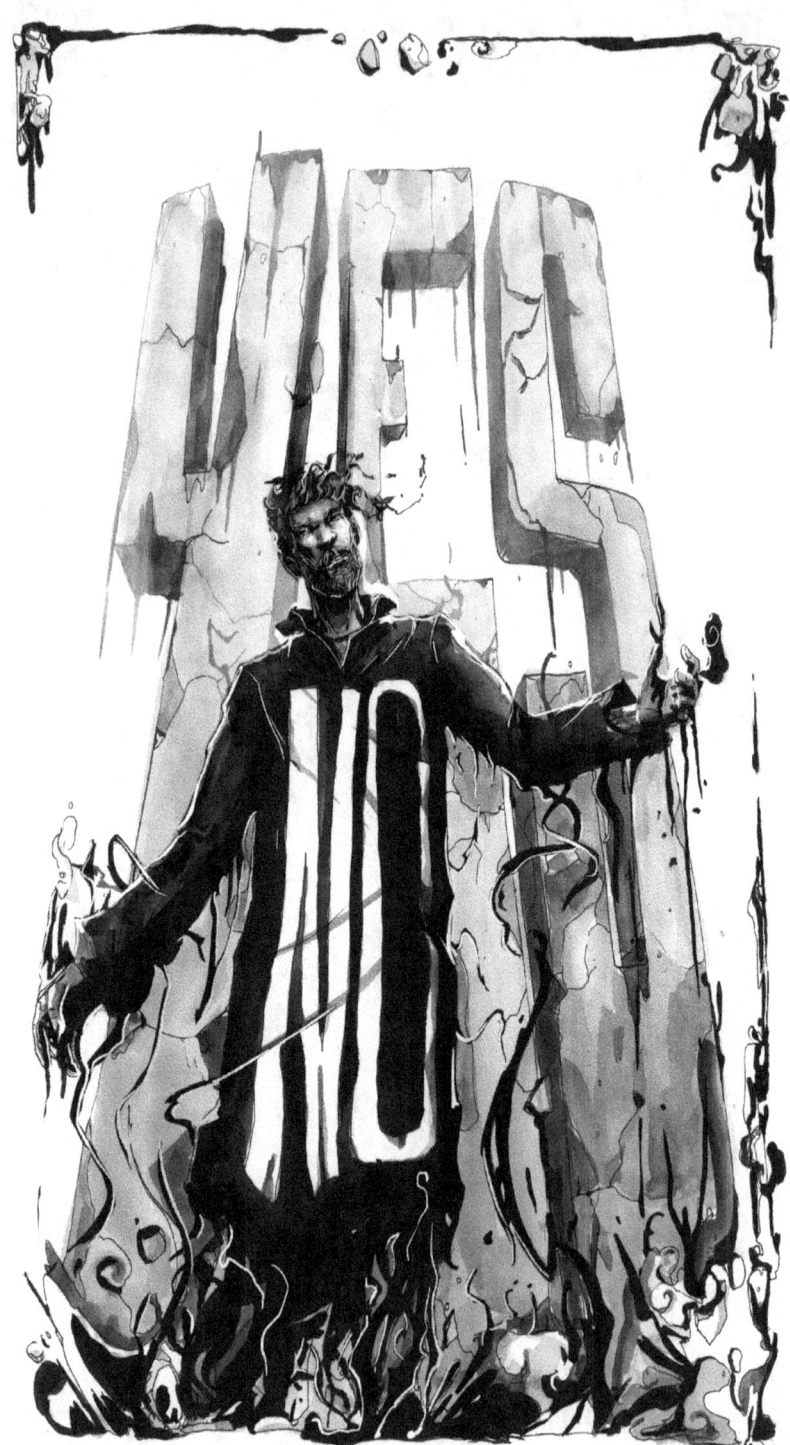

It's not enough to say yes to the things that matter most to you.

Yes is nothing without a no.

NO IS CRUCIAL TO CREATE THE CONDITIONS FOR A STATE OF FLOW—REMOVE THE UNNECESSARY, THE DISTRACTING, AND THE TRIVIAL.

Say no to the unimportant and the malicious little things that matter least, which feed on your time and leave nothing for the things that matter most.

By saying no, you are saying yes to focus, to productivity, to mastery.

A dramatic family member calling you to gossip and engage you in a toxic conversation that will drain you and ruin your day. No.

An unplanned meeting to discuss how to organize and clean the office fridge when a big project is underway. No.

A sales call. No.

Clearing out your emails because you committed to an inbox-zero challenge. No.

Reorganizing your closet because you couldn't find your favorite shirt. No.

With every no, you're saying yes to more time, better focus, joy, fulfillment, and higher energy. You're saying yes to what matters most to you, to getting important shit done, and to making a real difference in your life.

TEST

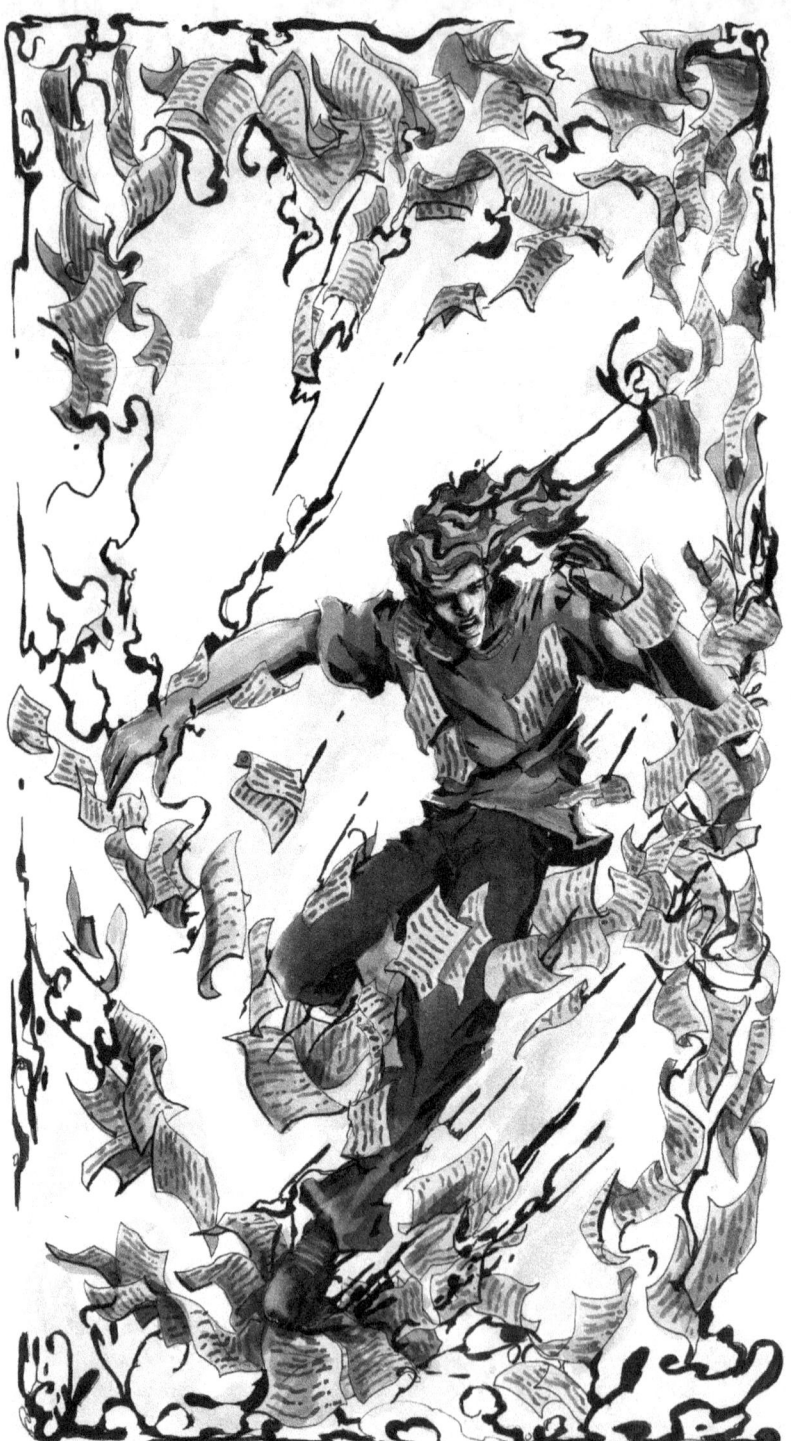

There are hundreds if not thousands of books on time management and productivity. Thousands more about all kinds of life advice and self-help.

Many offer brilliant ideas with real-world impact.

Some will work for you; others won't. The best way to know is to put them to the test.

BUT IF YOU DO NOT HAVE A STRATEGY AND A TESTING METHODOLOGY, YOU MAY END UP WITH UNWANTED CONSEQUENCES, AND YOU MAY EVEN DAMAGE WHATEVER GOOD THING YOU HAVE GOING.

CURB YOUR ENTHUSIASM

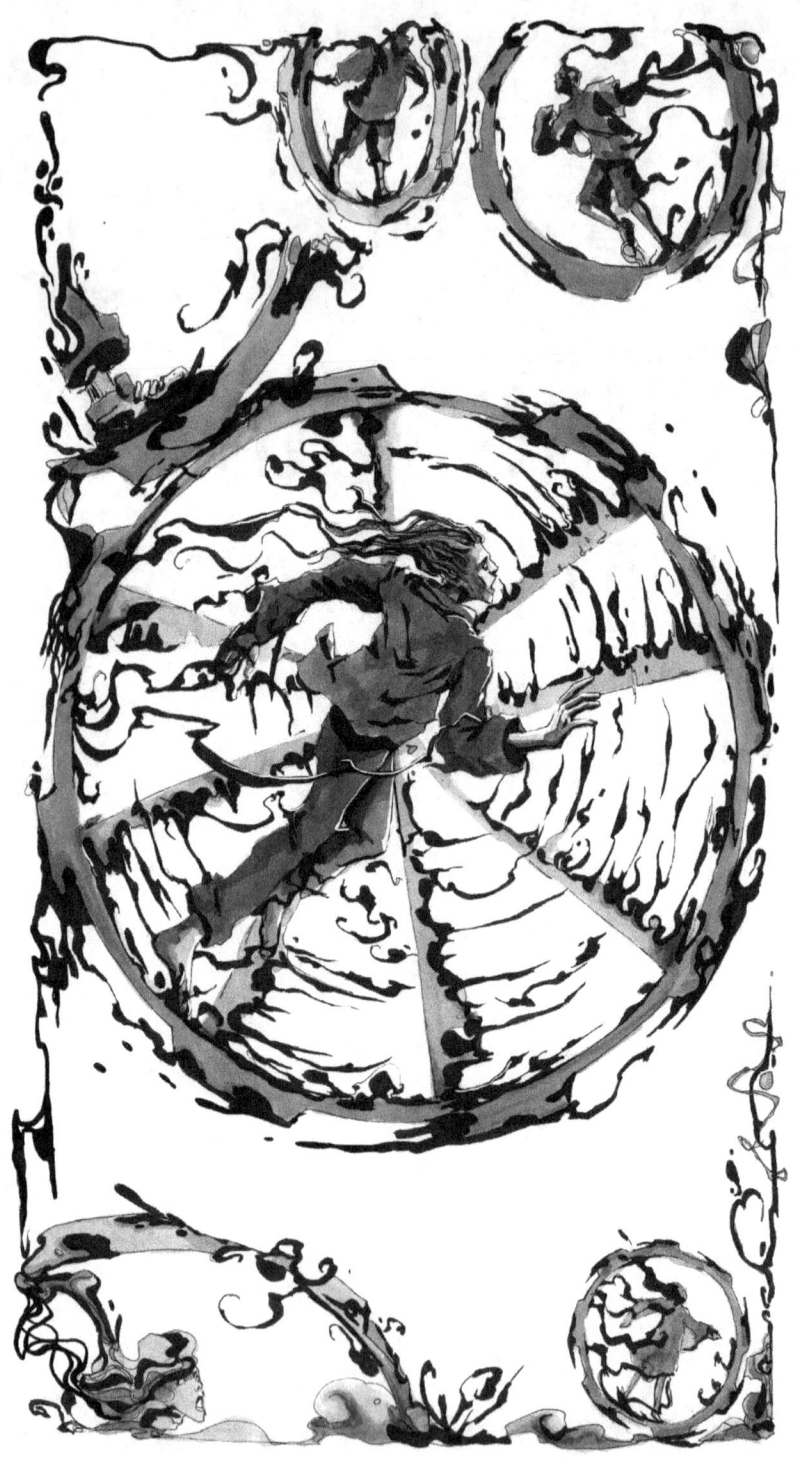

When reading a good book about the latest time management method or life hack, you will most likely get excited. The author makes sense, and he's prescribing what seems to be the perfect solution to the challenges you are facing.

Unfortunately, like most people, you may feel the need and build up the desire to change everything.

You convince yourself it's time.

You throw away the old because, of course, the new method can only work if applied in its totality.

You clear the slate, make preparations, and get started on Monday.

But your life has momentum, which progressively slows things down. Things and people around you don't adhere to your new way of doing things. They resist and cause friction.

By Thursday, you're in damage-control mode; you lean into your trusted old habits and work through the weekend to get things back on track by next Monday.

Another unrealistic book, another week lost, maybe what you have now is the best you can do.

It's not.

START WITH 20

WHEN YOU KNOW BETTER YOU DO BETTER

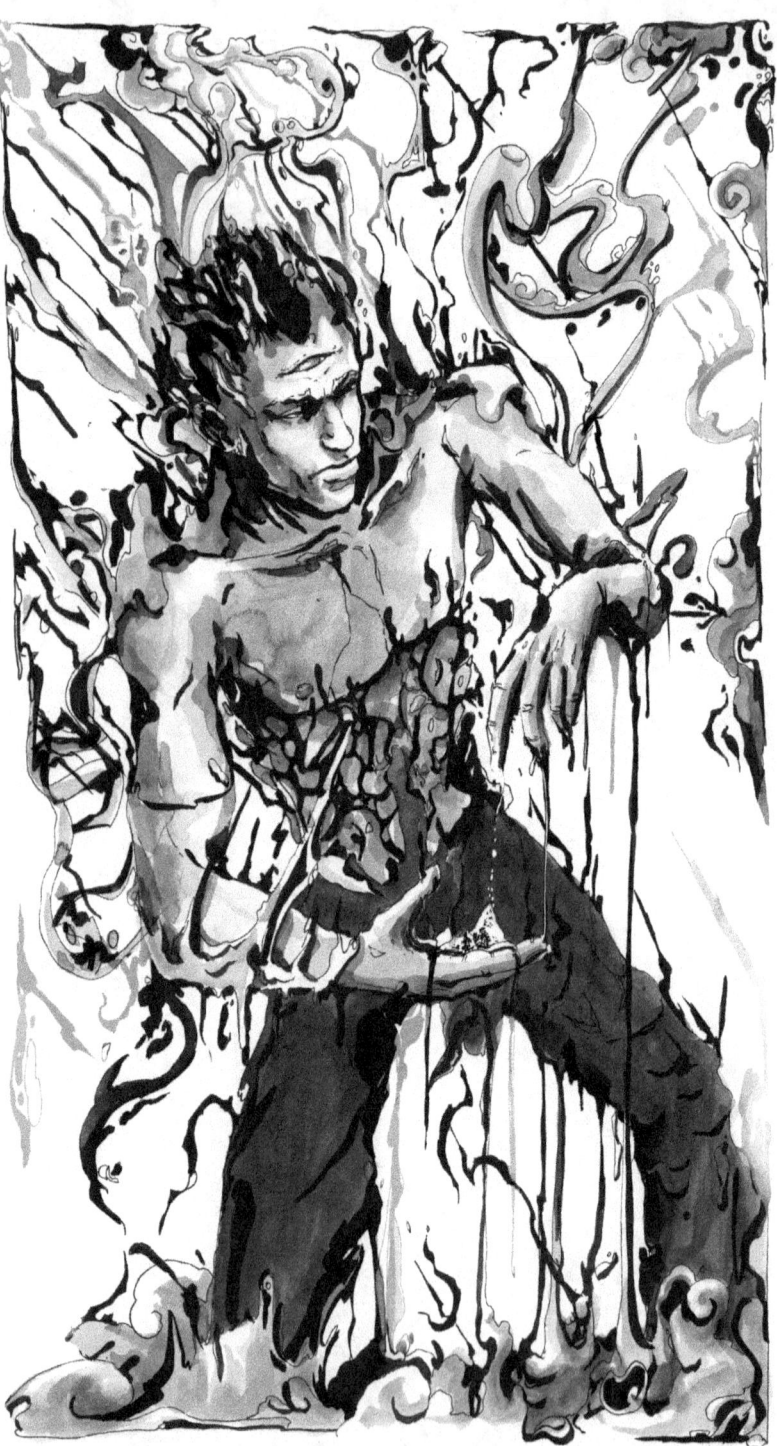

It's evolutionary, not revolutionary.

Changing everything will likely cause a significant reduction in your productivity and effectiveness. It will set your timelines back, driving you away further from your desired destination.

That is not to mention the impact on your state as you experience the results of your decision.

And in the end, you consume time to read about, test, and implement numerous time management strategies. Forget 100 percent. Start with 20 percent.

Use a maximum of 20 percent of your time and your workload, and use it to test new ways of doing things.

TAKE IT EASY, MAKE IT FUN, AND JAM ON IT.

Give it time, change it up, and make it work with your lifestyle and your schedule.

Think of yourself as the stress tester. You are not the guinea pig.

It's as if the author assigned you the task of testing his method and seeing when it breaks and what its limitations are.

See how far you can stretch and bend it. How easy and fast it is to apply it.

Estimate how much real impact it can have on your productivity, your life, and the one thing that matters most.

CHECK YOUR INTERNAL COMPASS.

Make your decision.

Move forward.

JAM ON IT

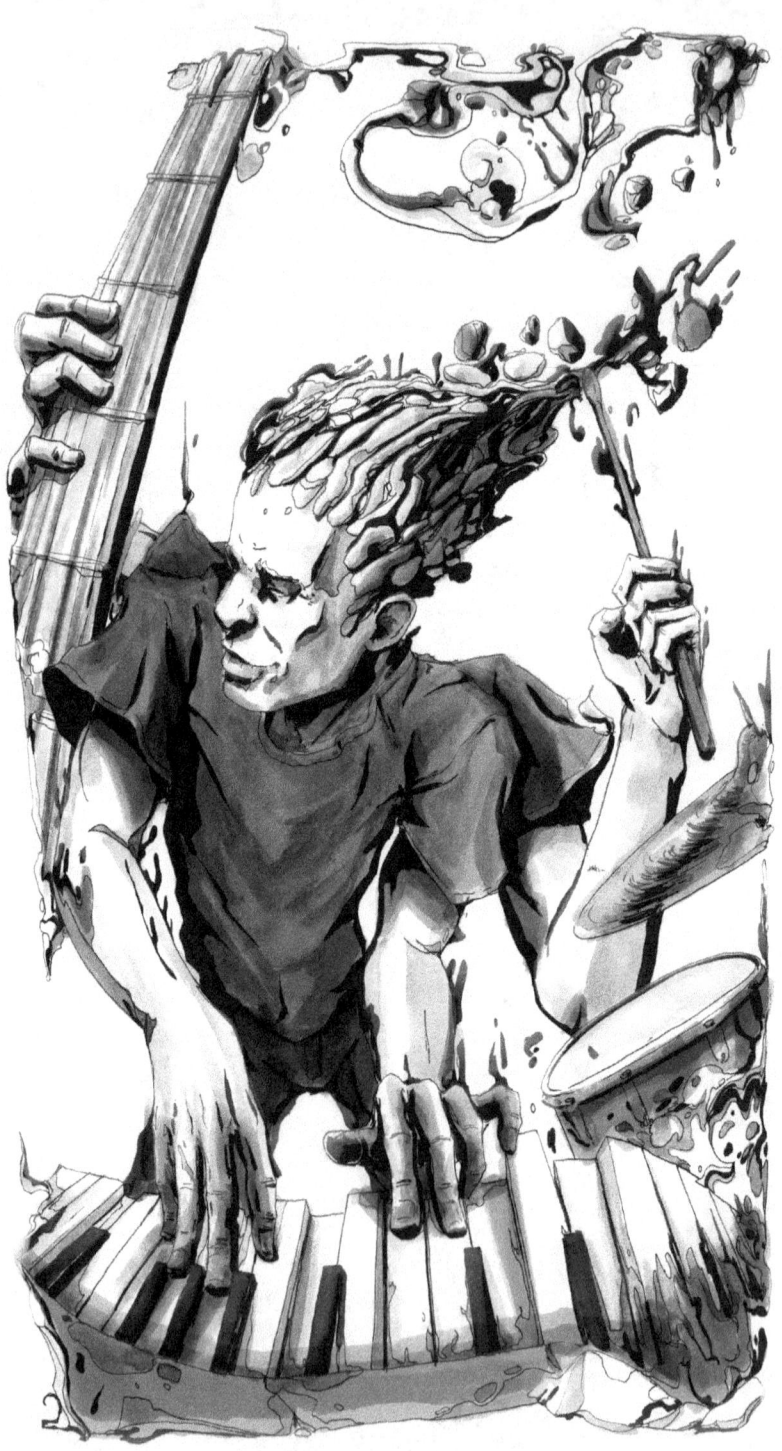

What if life was a series of jam sessions?

You are continually deciding who to jam with, what instruments to play, the music, the lyrics, the style, and whether or not guests are allowed.

You stop thinking about things in terms of right and wrong.

It's just a jam session!

It's not really about what you're doing as much as about what you want out of each jam session.

Sometimes it's about creating a hit pop single.

You choose people with relevant skills, modern instruments, upbeat rhythms, cheerful chord progression, and everything else to increase the likelihood of creating a hit.

At times it's just about having some fun, and it doesn't matter to you what comes out of the jam session.

So you choose people you love to be around, and nothing else matters.

Many times it's about more than one thing.

Maybe you want to create a great hit and have fun at the same time.

The brilliant thing about jam session decision-making is you can always have another go at it.

If a jam session doesn't go as intended and you are not happy with the outcome, you end it, change things up, and hold another jam session.

Then you hold another, and another, and another, until you get the outcome you want.

You simply experiment with different people, different instruments, and different styles, one jam session at a time.

The jam session decision-making process forces you to think about the outcome first.

AN EXPERIMENTAL APPROACH TO LIFE PUTS YOU IN CONTROL AND KEEPS YOU FOCUSED AND PRESENT.

Once you're clear on the outcome you want from the jam session, you are the one responsible for choosing the elements in such a way as to get the outcome you are after.

The more jam sessions you do, the more you learn about what works best and what can get you the results you want.

Whether you're happy with particular styles or you are into making every moment unique and different, the jam session approach gives you unlimited options. It becomes a powerful and flexible framework to discover fast, fun, effective, and enjoyable ways to achieve objectives.

Claim your decision-making superpowers.

UNSTOPPABLE

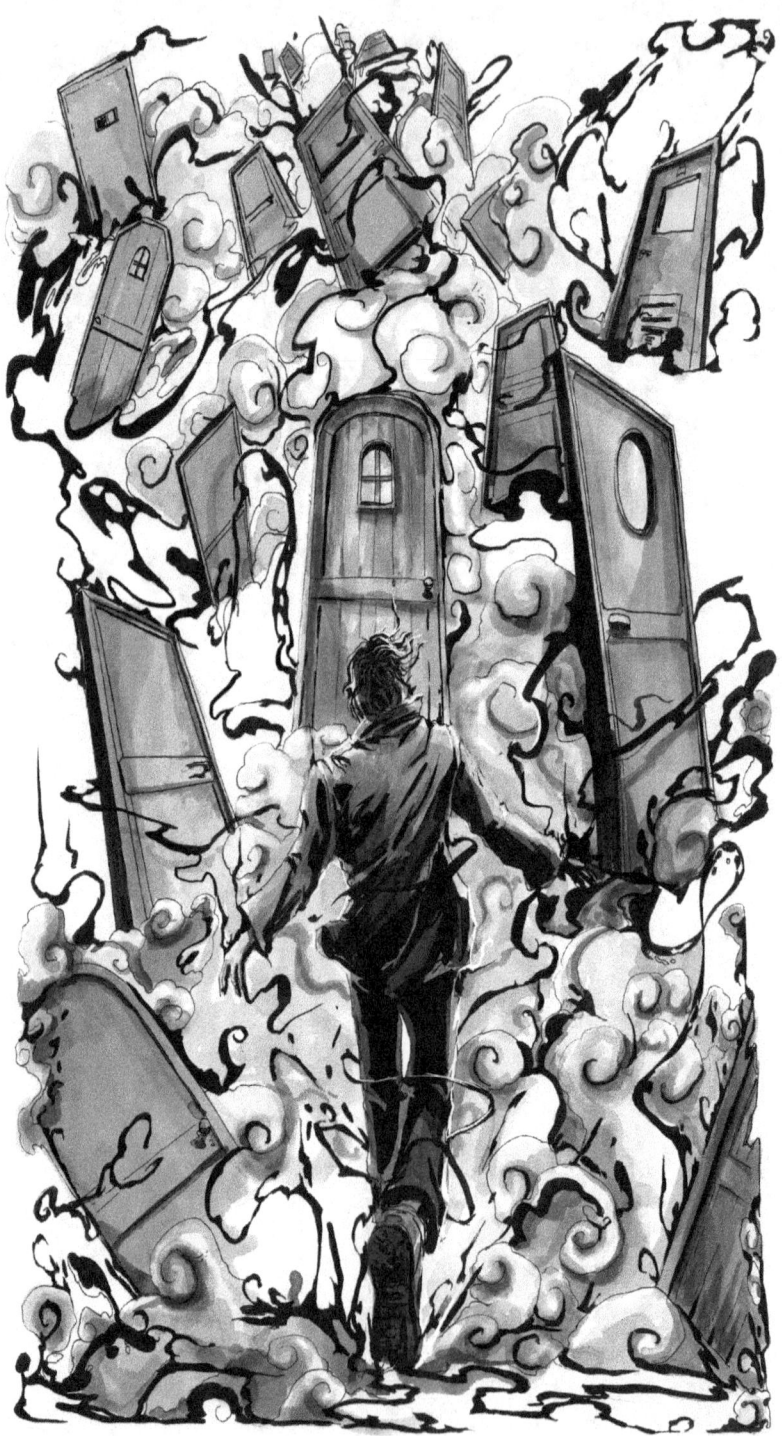

No one has all the answers, but many pretend they do, and they are all full of shit.

Even if they did, imagine living a life with nothing new to learn, no thrill, and no surprise!

Fuck answers. Questions are the shit.

Questions have the power to shape your life, guide you through the toughest of times, and open the doors to a universe of discovery.

A QUESTION HAS THE POWER OF A MILLION ANSWERS.

FASTER.
EASIER.
BETTER.

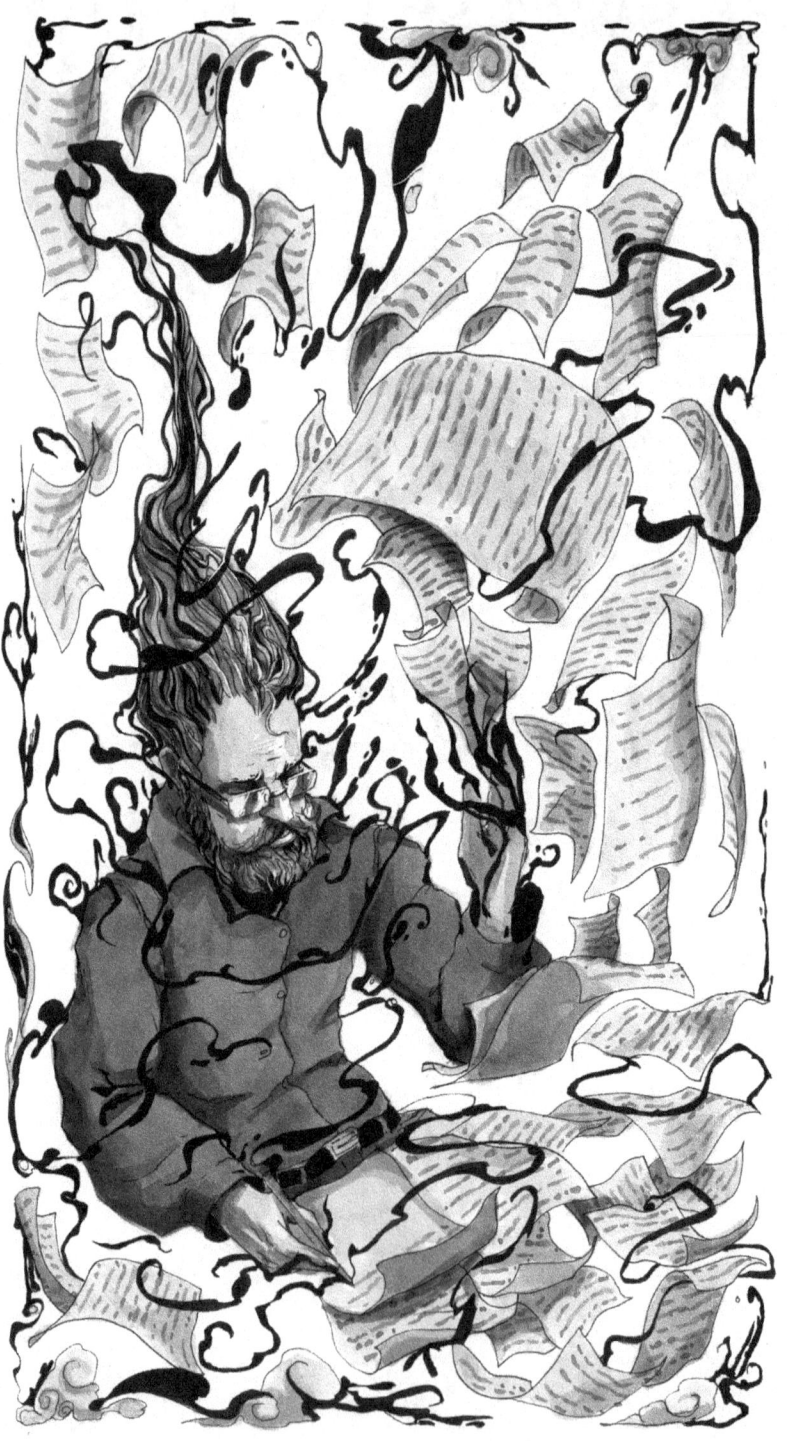

When you are faced with any challenge, obstacle, or barrier, your first inclination is to look for the best solution. The better way. The right answer.

That's the ultimate recipe for mediocracy.

If you want to be faster.

If you want things to be easier.

If you want to do better.

You must unleash the unstoppable power of human curiosity in you.

USE QUESTIONS TO MAKE BETTER CHOICES, TAKE MASSIVE ACTION, AND FOCUS YOUR ENERGY ON WHAT MATTERS MOST.

WHAT IS ENOUGH?

NOTHING IS, EVER

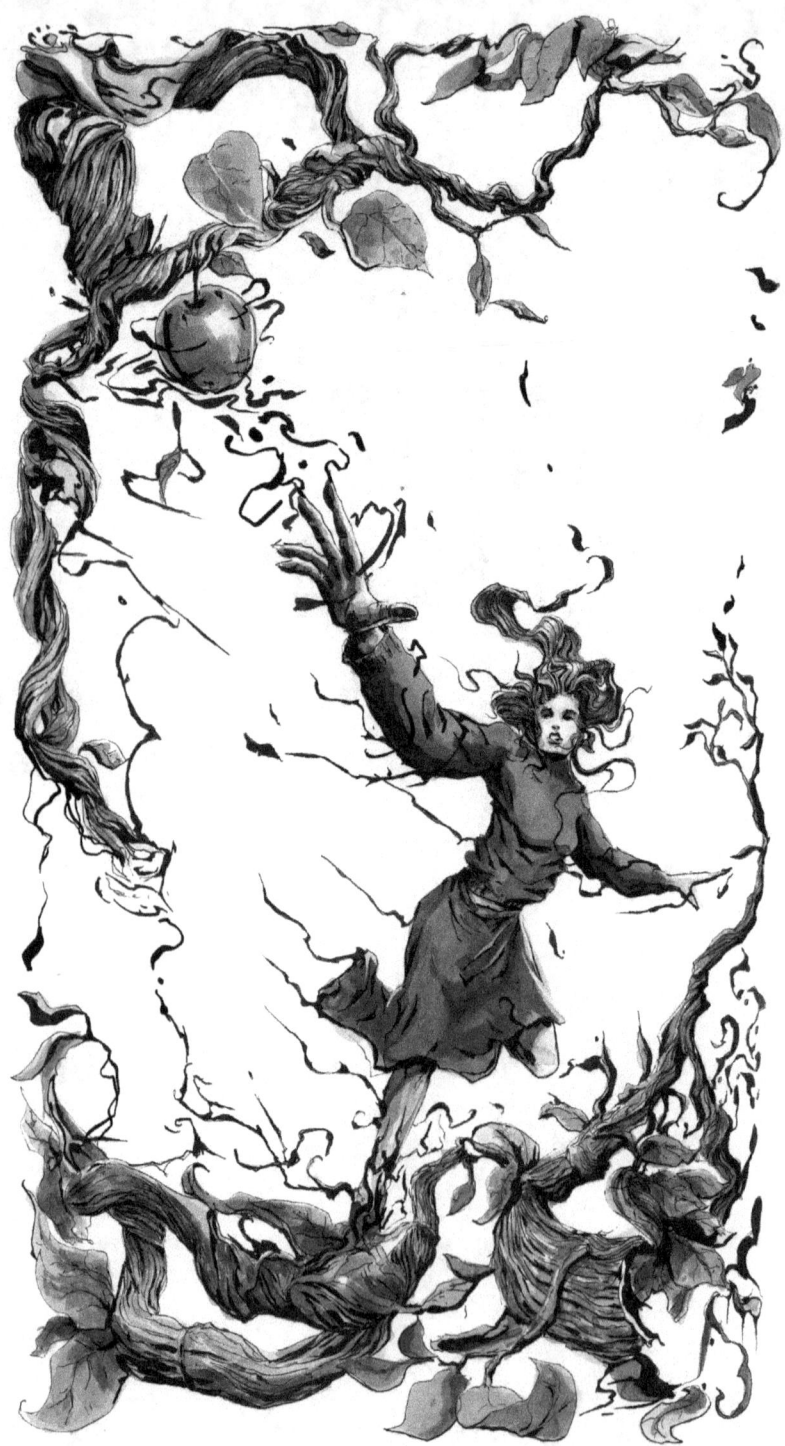

Growing up in Damascus, Syria, my family was well off, and my grandfather was wealthy.

But as things changed, I witnessed the depletion of my grandfather's fortune and the impact of the Syrian economic stagnation on our finances.

By the mid-1980s we were a poor family with a middle-income I. My parents wondered daily how they were going to pay for things and who they were going to reach out to next to borrow some money to make ends meet.

Through it all, their generosity remained strong. Our home was not just ours; it was for an endless stream of guests, friends, family members, distant cousins, anyone in town for a couple of days, even an old neighbor from ten years ago, and students from Mom's special needs school.

Visitors stayed hours on end and stayed over for days; no one would wonder why this person was eating our food or using our stuff.

For me, each new person was a fresh victim! I'd bring out my toys and start showcasing how awesome and noisy they were—so many fire trucks and police cars. In later years, I'd showcase my drawings and then my guitar playing. Poor souls,

I think my parents owed them food and shelter for surviving me!

Our home came alive with people.

Yes, we had to split our food with them.

Yes, I was inconvenienced every time I had to run out to get more food.

And yes, my parents had to figure out how to get more money.

But we had a happy, joyous home.

THERE WAS A REAL SENSE OF BELONGING, A SENSE THAT PEOPLE HAD EACH OTHER'S BACKS, ENJOYED EACH OTHER'S PRESENCE, AND SOMEHOW THERE WAS ALWAYS ENOUGH TO GO AROUND.

Funny enough, at the same time, many with far more money and more resources had far fewer people who wanted to be around them or in their company.

So what is enough?

I realized that nothing is. Not unless you choose it to be so.

For me, I love that perpetual state of hunger. So in a way, nothing is ever enough.

LIFE IS REMARKABLE, SO WHY NOT HAVE MORE OF EVERYTHING?!

CHOICE

YOUR LIFE YOUR WAY

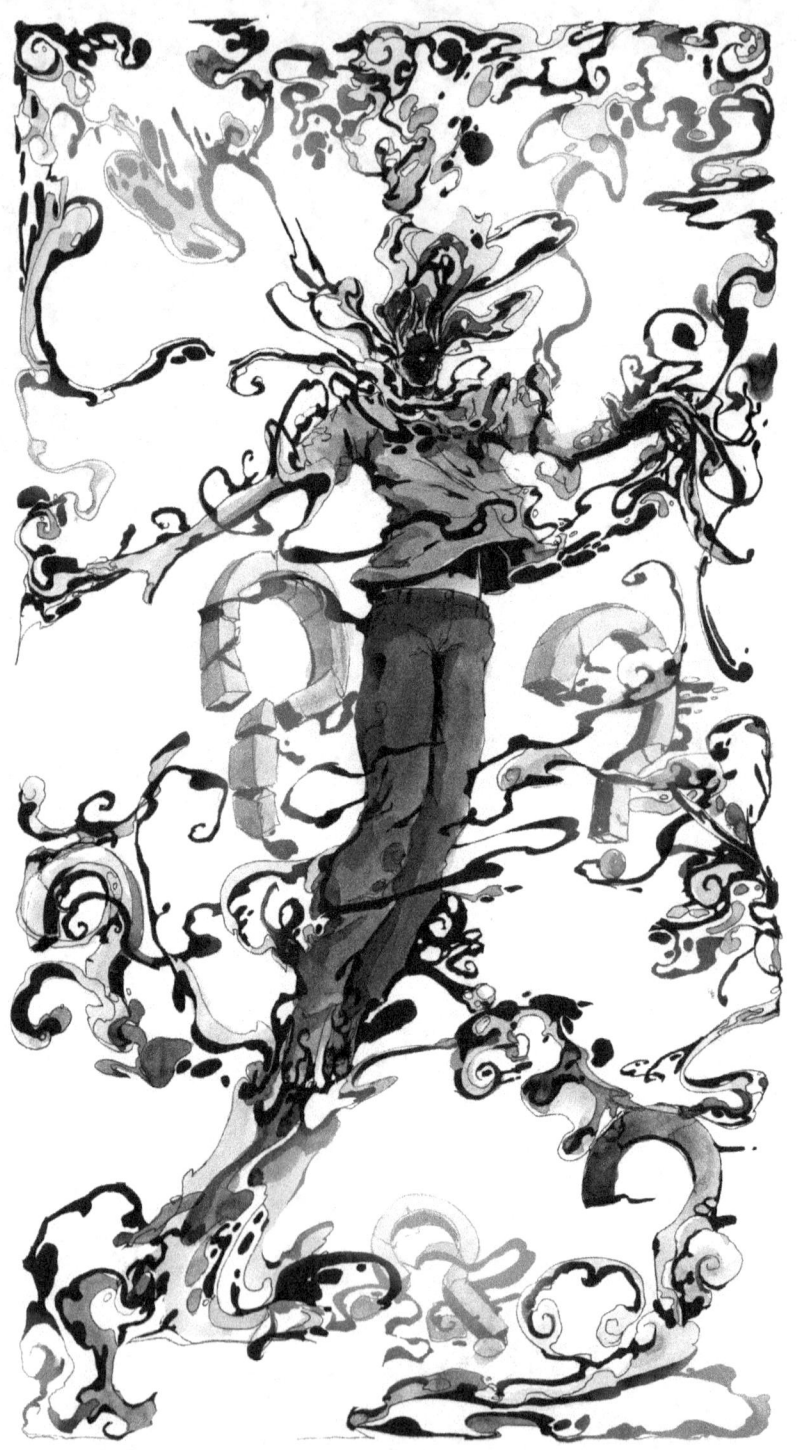

Instead of focusing on *what* is enough, getting curious about *why* something is enough and *why* it isn't will lead you down the path of fulfillment and the power of choice.

Instead of satisfying desires you've dreamt up based on what you learned should be enough, you can choose to go after what truly fulfills you.

To me, it's the unplanned weekend walk with my eleven-year-old daughter versus the perfectly planned family trip at a tropical resort.

A few no-agenda meetings with random people who reach out asking for help, versus a keynote at a world conference.

Advising a local startup, versus consulting with a multimillion-dollar corporation.

What is it for you?

I am still very much human with an insatiable hunger for position, influence, power, attention, and spotlight, and from time to time I indulge in it.

But for my everyday life nourishment, I rigorously stick to a course of love, dipped in relationships, and seasoned with giving back. That's enough for me.

What's enough for you?

And why?

IT'S NOT ABOUT RIGHT OR WRONG. IT'S ABOUT CHOICE, DISCOVERY, AND MAKING SURE YOU'RE GOING AFTER WHAT MATTERS MOST. LIVE YOUR LIFE, YOUR WAY, RIGHT HERE AND RIGHT FUCKIN' NOW.

THIS BOOK IS IMPOSSIBLE

A THANK YOU

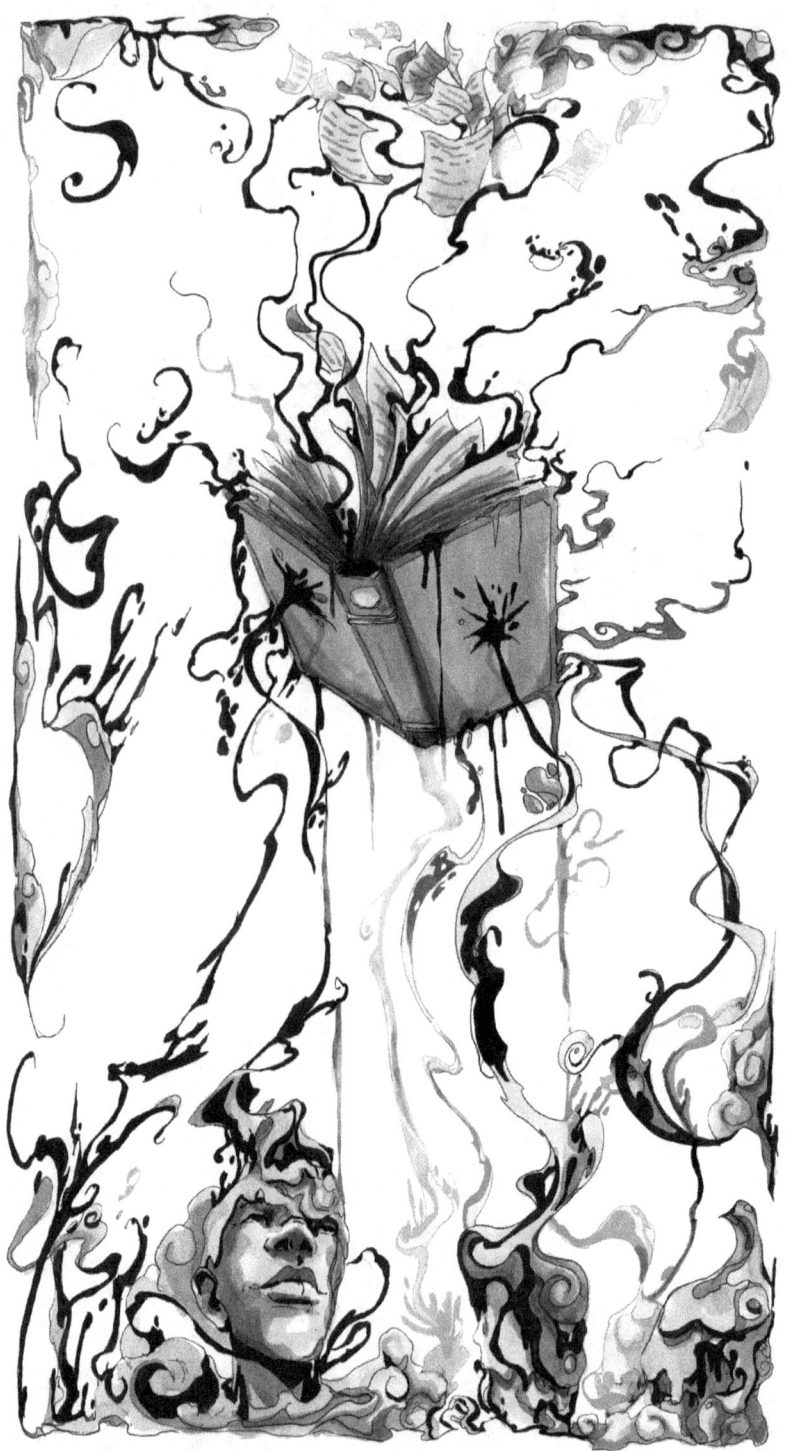

Like anything worth doing in life, this book is impossible. If it wasn't for family, friends, mentors, coaches, supporters, and allies.

Rama, the love of my life who believed in me, invested in me, stood by me for twenty years of ups and downs, and is still here for me with every sunrise, making my life worth living.

My remarkable mom, Fatima, in many ways that I can never count, made me the person I am today, pushed me to be better, and gave her all selflessly to our family.

Hassan, my late dad, from whom I got my love for reading, writing, and poetry, learned empathy, love, and standing for what I believe in.

My siblings Laila and Hamod, for tolerating me while growing up, trying to figure out who I am, and being there when our family was in need. You were unwitting allies who gave me the space to focus on building my life.

Zain, my eldest, for the thoughtful and engaging conversations. I have to pinch myself to remember you are still a teen every time we talk.

Julie, my youngest, for the never-ending spring of love, care, joy, and surprise that makes every day worth living.

Joel Mark Harris, Sam Thiara, Tristram Waye, Vis Naidoo, Sarah Al Marashi, Cameron Brown, thank you for helping me even when I didn't ask, generously giving your time and energy, and being honest with your input and feedback. You are a positive force in my life, and I'm a much better version of myself because of you.

LIFE DOES NOT BOOK APPOINTMENTS.

YOU CAN'T STOP LIFE, CAN'T SLOW IT DOWN, AND YOU CAN'T HOLD ON TO IT. BUT YOU CAN MASTER IT.

ABOUT THE AUTHOR

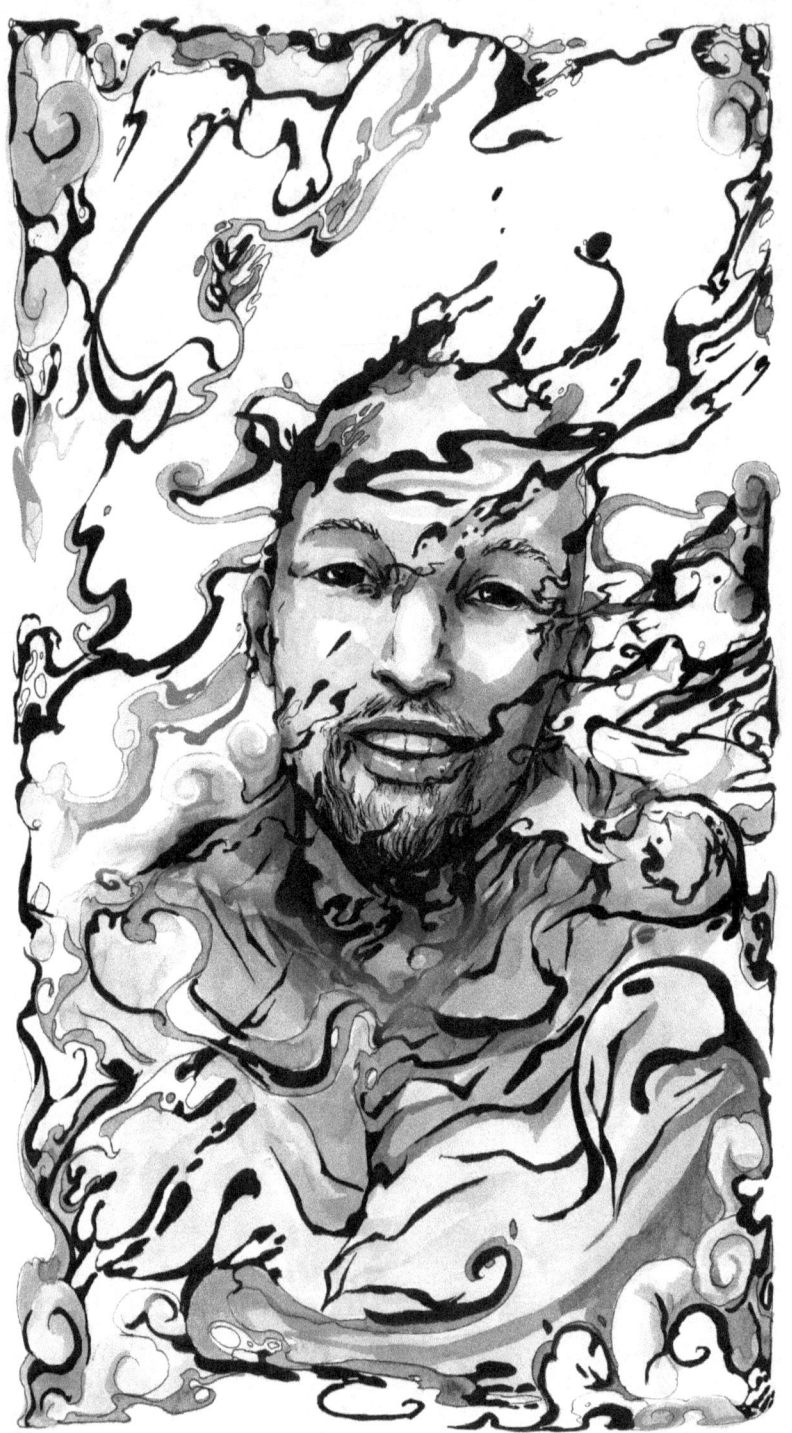

Syrian-born Canadian troublemaker, clueless father, hopeless romantic, and people person. Recovering engineer and tech geek, builder of things that sometimes work.

Closeted neat freak, easygoing, coffee-loving thinker. Politics addict, social justice advocate, highly opinionated bookworm, dedicated follower of the cult of science.

Vaccinated child of a caring mother, masked during pandemics, flat earth denier, global warming fact believer.

Lifelong learner.

www.ingramcontent.com/pod-product-compliance
Lightning Source LLC
Chambersburg PA
CBHW070132080526
44586CB00015B/1664